POSTMENOPAUSAL HEART AND BONE HEALTH

Empowering Women To Take Charge Of Their Health By Adopting Healthy Lifestyles For A Vibrant Life Beyond Menopause.

DR. DINESH KANFADE

ACKNOWLEDGEMENTS

I wish to express my gratitude to various sources, knowingly or unknowingly has contributed for empowering my knowledge, empowering women's health and helping me to write this book.

I would like to thank my mentors and teachers who had been a torch bearer for me for writing this book.

I also express my sincere gratitude to my family members and friends who have always been supportive and motivated me in my initiatives in writing series of books on **"Women's Health"**, this book being third in the series.

DEDICATION

Dedicated to my better half Nita,

son Akshay, daughter-in-law Priya

and little sweet Avni.

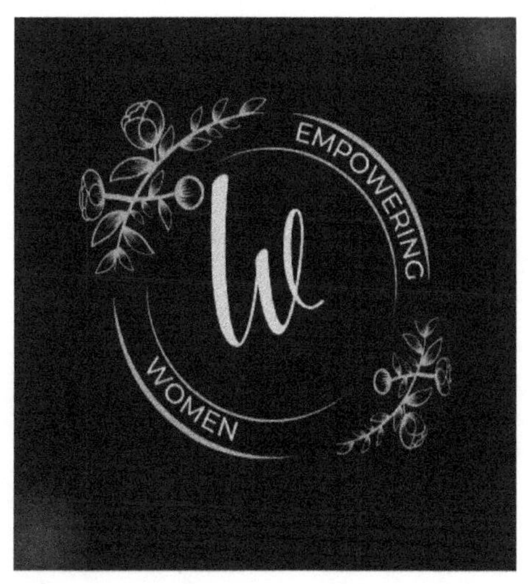
EMPOWERING
WOMEN

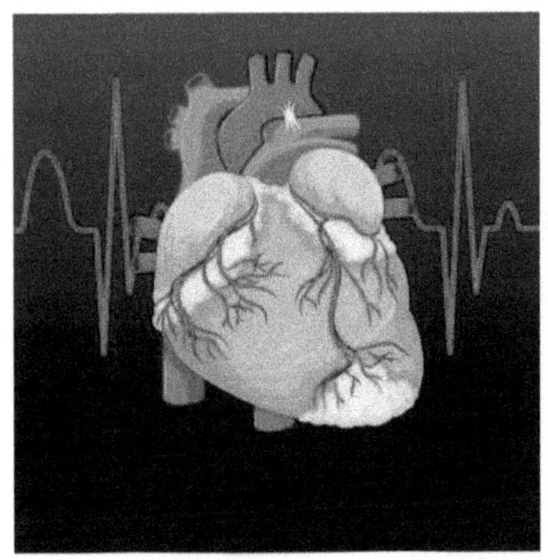

Source: Freepik.com

"We can no longer ignore heart disease. While awareness is important, it's time for women to take action now – to love and protect their hearts by maintaining healthy lifestyles"

Karen Murray

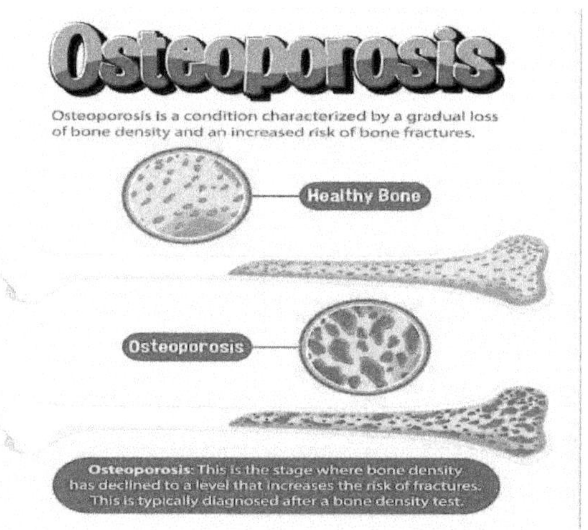

Source: Freepik.com

"Osteoporosis is not an inevitable part of ageing, it is preventable. So it is vital that all of us, of all ages, start taking care of our bones now before it is too late."

Camilla Parker Bowles

FOREWORD

As I stand on the threshold of introducing you this remarkable book, **"Postmenopausal Heart and Bone Health"** I am filled with a sense of privilege and excitement. Having had the opportunity to witness the evolution of this project, I am humbled by the dedication, passion, and expertise that the author has poured into every page.

In this ageing world, where women's health topics are sometimes overlooked or underestimated, this book serves as a beacon of knowledge and empowerment. It's a guide for postmenopausal women seeking to take charge of their heart and bone health, and it's also a tribute to the resilience and strength that define this phase of life.

With great anticipation, I invite you to delve into **"Postmenopausal Heart and Bone Health"** and discover the remarkable insights that lie within.

This book should be read by the concerned healthcare providers, medical students and the women of all age groups.

My best wishes for his future endeavors.

Dr. Uday Jogalekar

Sr. Obstetrician & Gynecologist

IVF Specialist

Director, Abhyuday Maternity & Nursing Home, Virar

PREFACE

The greatest achievement of the last century is greater longevity that has resulted in aged population worldwide. The advantage of increased longevity is only when it is translated into healthy ageing. It is obvious that women live significant part of their life after menopause. Many women going through menopause experience unpleasant symptoms such as hot flushes, night sweats, anxiety, depression and poor sleep which can affect their relationship with their spouse. Additionally, the risk of non-communicable diseases such as cardiovascular disease, osteoporosis, hypertension, diabetes and cancer increase after menopause.

In the pages that follow, we embark on a journey to explore the intricate interplay between **the heart and bone health in the lives of postmenopausal women**. This book is a culmination of extensive research, thoughtful analysis, and a deep commitment for shedding light on the vital aspects of women's health during this significant phase of life.

As women go through menopause transition, they experience a myriad of changes that can impact their cardiovascular health and bone density. Estrogen deficiency in menopausal women pose additional risk factor in the causation of heart disease and osteoporosis other than the conventional risk factors common to both genders due to ageing. Our aim is to unravel the complexities of these connections, providing a comprehensive understanding that empowers both women and healthcare professionals alike.

To the readers embarking on this exploration, your curiosity and dedication for understanding these critical health aspects are commendable. As we journey together through the pages ahead; you may find inspiration, knowledge and a renewed sense of agency over your heart and bone health.

Dr. Dinesh Kanfade

Sr. Obstetrician & Gynecologist

Life Member Indian Menopause Society

TABLE OF CONTENTS:

CHAPTER I: INTRODUCTION

"Women with heart and bone health are intertwined, as cardiovascular disease and osteoporosis pose significant risk. Taking proactive steps to protect both is crucial for a healthy and vibrant life".

Dr. Jane Doe

(A) Why cardiovascular disease and osteoporosis need to be taken seriously?

As per the CDC Report (Centre for Disease Control and Prevention):

- Despite an increase in awareness over the past decades, only about half (56%) of women recognize that heart disease is their number one killer, cancer being second.

- Heart is the leading cause of death for women in United States, killing 314186 women in 2020: or about 1 in every 5 female deaths.

- Although heart disease was initially thought of as a man's disease, almost as many women as men die of heart disease each year in menopausal age group in United States.

As per the research studies:

- Osteoporotic fractures are known to generate a heavy burden of morbidity, mortality and financial risk.
- Fractures particularly of spines and hip pose the most serious complications.
- Despite improvement in the treatment of hip fracture patients, only 60% recover all their previous functions. Between 7.9 and 26.9 % die within 3 to 6 months and 25% have levels of disability that require constant care throughout life.

(B) Greater Longevity:

- We are living in ageing world. Women have to live significant part of their life after menopause. Menopause itself is not a disease. It is completely a natural ageing event in women's life.
- Because menopause occurs later in life, it is challenging to separate the increased risk of non-communicable diseases due to ageing and increased risk due to menopause. The biology and symptomatology of menopause is blurred due to its relationship to the underlying ageing process. **However several studies have shown that long term effects on the heart and bone health are related to estrogen deficiency.**

- Globally **life expectancy** has increased from 66.5 to 73.5 years in between 2000 to 2019, while **healthy life expectancy** has increased from 58.3 to 63.5 years. It clearly means that **healthy life expectancy (5.4)** is not keeping pace with the **life expectancy (6.6),** meaning thereby 1.2 years lived in disability. All countries irrespective of their state of economic development face an increasing burden of non-communicable diseases.

(C) Few questionnaire for you:

- Are you aware of the hidden risks that lurk within menopausal years?

- Are you aware of the fact that some women have nontraditional risk factors for cardiovascular disease in addition to the menopause transition and ageing risk?

- Do you know that cardiovascular disease is the number one killer in women?

- Do you know that 80% of the cardiovascular events can be prevented with healthy eating and physical activities?

- Do you know that osteoporosis is not an inevitable part of ageing and healthy lifestyle including diet rich in calcium and vitamin D, also the physical activities can prevent it?

(D) Story of a vibrant and independent woman:

To answer above questions, I will have to narrate here the story of a vibrant and independent woman named Nita. She has recently entered the postmenopausal stage of her life and was enjoying the newfound freedom it brought. Because by the time her children were grown up and taking higher education, she has her own home, her husband was also well settled in his business. However Nita soon began to look changes in her body that concerned her.

One day while walking in the park, Nita stumbled and fell, fracturing her wrist. She had been to healthcare professional for treatment of fracture, did some investigations as per the advice, realized that her bone density is too low and that's why she **sustained fracture with a lesser trauma.** Determined to take control of her health, Nita started researching the importance of bone health in postmenopausal women.

As she delve deeper into her research, Nita discovered that osteoporosis, a condition characterized by weakened bones, was a common concerned for women in her age group. She learned that the declined estrogen level during menopause can accelerate bone loss, putting women at higher risk of fracture and other complications.

Motivated to protect her bones, Nita began incorporating weight-bearing exercises such as walking, jogging and strength training, into her daily routine. She also made sure to consume a balanced diet rich in calcium and vitamin D, essential nutrients for bone health.

But Nita's journey didn't stop here. As she continued her quest for knowledge, she came to know another fact: postmenopausal women are also at an increased risk of developing cardiovascular disease. This revelation made her realize the importance of taking care of her heart as well.

Nita started paying more attention to her cardiovascular health by adopting heart-friendly habits. She quit her smoking, reduced her intake of processed food high in saturated fats and started incorporating more fruits, vegetables and whole grains in her diet. Regular exercises such as brisk walking and swimming became part of her routine too.

Over the time, Nita's dedication to heart and bone health paid off. She felt stronger, more energetic and confident in her ability to live a healthy life. By taking proactive steps to protect her heart and bones, Nita became inspiration to the other postmenopausal women in her community.

Nita's story serves as a lesson to remind the importance of heart and bone health in postmenopausal women. It highlights the need for awareness, education and proactive measures to maintain a healthy and vibrant life during this stage.

In the past, menopause may not have received as much attention due to variety of reasons.

One factor could be the cultural and social norms that placed less emphasis on women's health. Menopause was often taken as a natural part of ageing and not given much consideration beyond that.

Medications and lifestyle modifications for menopause that can help alleviate discomfort and perhaps prevent or delay the onset of non-communicable diseases such as cardiovascular disease and osteoporosis, have been around the decades in various forms. But research indicates that just a minority of menopausal women are receiving the medical care they deserve.

Women today are more empowered to speak up about their health concerns and seek information and support. **The availability of book like this,** the online resources, support groups and healthcare professionals who specialize in menopause has also contributed in the increased awareness.

The International menopause society (established in 1970) in collaboration with World Health Organization **(WHO)** has designated **October 18 as "World Menopause Day"** and the month as **"Menopause Awareness Month".** The global initiatives are dedicated to millions of mature women of 40 plus who are going to spend one third of their life after menopause and are unaware or ignorant about the positive steps to be taken for improving their quality of life in the second inning – the postmenopausal life. Indian menopause society (established in 1995) with its member societies are trying hard to sensitize the healthcare professionals especially the practicing gynecologist towards the health of post-menopausal women.

This is my humble attempt to revisit menopause and I hope that the healthcare professionals will promote menopausal care and counseling. I will also appeal women to come out of the age-cage and redefine age for graceful life ahead.

Cameron Diaz has rightly said:

"My belief is that it's privilege to get older. Not everybody gets to get older".

Before going into the depth of heart and bone health in menopausal women, I will like to describe the pathophysiology and symptomatology of menopause in short in the next chapter.

CHAPTER II: PATHOPHYSIOLOGY AND SYMPTOMATOLOGY OF MENOPAUSE

"Menopause is inevitable.

But one can make it easy and equally

beautiful by understanding it."

(A) Definition:

- Menopause is defined by Stedman as permanent cessation of menses. An awareness of menopause can be traced from ancient Greeks. In fact, the word menopause is derived from the Greek word 'meno' meaning month and refers to menstrual cycle, while 'pause' meaning to cease or to stop. In other words menopause literally means cessation of monthly cycles.

- The World Health Organization **(WHO)** has defined natural menopause as the permanent cessation of menses resulting from loss of ovarian follicular activity. Menopause marks the end of reproductive life and natural menopause is the retrospective clinical diagnosis which occurs after 12 consecutive months of amenorrhoea, for which no other pathological cause can be established.

- The menopausal transition is the time before the final menopausal period (FMP) and is associated with irregular cycles, hormonal instability and symptoms.

(B) Pathophysiology of menopause transition:

- **Biology of ovarian aging:**
  In the human ovary, there is a continuous and progressive decline in the number of follicles from foetal life onwards. From several million follicles present at birth, less than a thousand remain at menopause. The loss cannot be accounted for by ovulation alone. Because the reproductive span of 30-35 years in a woman can only account for a loss of 350-450 ovarian follicles through ovulation. Their disappearance is also related to a loss of oocytes and surrounding granulosa and theca cells of the ovarian follicles that occur continuously through a process of follicular atresia. In every cycle, from a recruited pool of growing follicles, only one dominant follicle is selected, the rest undergoing atresia. It is clear from several studies (Block 1952, Gougeon 1984, Gosden 1985, Richardson et al 1987) that serum gonadotropins mainly follicular stimulating hormone (FSH) are responsible for accelerating the pace of follicular atresia leading to the depletion of stock and subsequent menopause.

- **Menopause Markers (Hormonal Changes during menopause transition)**:
  The transition from the ovulatory cycles to the menopausal state is usually not an instantaneous event. Rather it is a series of hormonal clinical alterations that reflect declining ovarian function. Menopause is diagnosed retrospectively by history. Markers for diagnosis of menopause are preferably restricted for use in special situations and for fertility issues.

- **FSH** (Follicle Stimulating Hormone) > 10 IU/L is indicative of declining ovarian function.

- **FSH** > 20 IU/L is diagnostic of ovarian failure in the perimenopausal age group with vasomotor symptoms (VMS) even in the absence of complete cessation of menses.

- **FSH** > 40 IU/L done 2 months apart is diagnostic of menopause.

- **FSH** rise precedes the LH rise.

- **FSH** is a diagnostic marker of ovarian failure while LH is not.

- **LH** (Luteinizing Hormone) measurement is not necessary to make a diagnosis of menopause.

- 1 - 3 years after menopause, serum LH rises by 3 folds while FSH by 10 - 20 folds. Rise in serum LH level is less pronounced than serum FSH level because:

    - LH has a shorter half-life and has no specific negative feedback peptide.

    - FSH has a specific negative feedback peptide called Inhibin.

- Postmenopausal serum estradiol level falls and it is < 20 pg/ml at menopause. (Premenopausal level of serum estradiol varies from 40 -400 pg/ml)

- AMH and Inhibin levels are low or undetectable at menopause. Inhibin is a polypeptide that is secreted by granulosa cells, it has both paracrine and endocrine functions. At the central level, inhibin exerts a negative feedback effect and reduces the pituitary secretion of FSH. At the ovarian level its paracrine function is to prevent folliculogenesis of other follicles. **An increasing level of serum FSH during early follicular phase and a decline in circulating levels of inhibin and estradiol are the first indications of age-related acceleration of follicular depletion.** Serum inhibin during the early follicular phase showed a significant decline in women of 45-49 years of age as compared to those aged below 45 years (McLachlan et.al. 1987-88).

- On transvaginal ultrasound the antral follicular count is low and ovarian volume is also reduced.

- **Changes in cycle length and menstrual bleeding**:
  Women aged 18-24 years have an average follicular phase length of 15 ± 2 days, but those aged 40 -44 years have an average length of 10 + 2 days, which tends to shorten the menstrual cycle. Thus menstrual cycle length may shorten before it lengthens as women progress through the transition (Trealar et al 1967). One hallmark of the menopause transition is a change in bleeding pattern, Van Voorhis and Et. al. have studied hormonal pattern and menstrual bleeding pattern in a large sub cohort of the SWAN participants aged 42-52 years. They found that 20% of all cycles during the time were un-ovulatory. They also noted that short cycle lengths (<21 days) were common early in menopause transition whereas long cycle intervals (> 36 days) were associated with late menopause transition.

(C) Age at menopause:

- The menopause transition most often begins between ages 45 and 55 years. The average age at menopause of an Indian woman is 46.2 years, much less than western woman (51 years).

- From available Indian data it is hypothesized that an early age at menopause in Indian women (46.2 years) predisposes them to chronic health disorders a decade earlier than the Caucasians having late age at menopause (51 years).

- It is reported that osteoporotic fractures occur 10-20 years earlier in Indians as compared to Caucasians.

- The first myocardial infarction (MI) attack occurs in 4.4% of Asian women at a younger age than in European women.

- In India, type II diabetes occurs a decade earlier than the Caucasians.

- Breast cancer is the most common cancer in Indian women and the incidence peaks before the age of 50 years.

As the women approach their mid-forties, many women find themselves looking for signs of menopause and trying to figure out when it will begin for them. Most women reach menopause between the ages of 45 and 55 years. But as every woman is unique, age at menopause may also differ due to underlying conditions.

- **Genetic factors:**
  Research has conclusively shown that there is a strong link between menopause and genetics. There are approximately 50% chances that a woman will become menopausal at the same age as her mother or within a few years of that age. However, this may not always be the case.

- **Ethnicity:**
  Studies have conclusively revealed that the average menopausal age for Caucasian women in the UK and USA is around 51 years, while in Indians it is 46.2 yrs. The reason for these variations is that women of different ethnicities often have different levels of estrogenic activity.

- **Smoking**:
  Smoking has been found to be the number one modifiable lifestyle factor relating to early

menopause. Polycyclic aromatic hydrocarbons found in cigarette smoke are toxic to ovarian follicles. These chemicals can cause premature loss of follicles leading to early onset of menopause. Smoking can lead to faster breakdown of oestrogen in the liver which in turn results in an earlier decline in oestrogen level.

- **Body Mass Index (BMI)**:

  A study conducted by Australian University has shown that Women who are underweight or have a low BMI are more likely to enter menopause early, while women who are overweight or have high BMI are more likely to experience a late menopause. This is due to the fact that oestrogen is stored in fat cells.

- **Parity**:

  Nulliparous women may experience an earlier menopause while multiparty or a late first pregnancy may result in a later onset.

- **Other factors include:**

- Women with bilateral oophorectomy, exposure to radiotherapy or chemotherapy in premenopausal age experiencing early induced menopause.

- Use of oral contraceptives may delay the onset.

Is there a menopause age calculator?
All factors discussed above could help women to determine the appropriate age at menopause but there

is no definite test to predict it. In a nutshell AMH levels indicate the number of follicles present in the ovaries and unlike FSH levels, AMH levels do not fluctuate with phases in menstrual cycles, which means that they can be used to determine the extent of ovarian reserve and thereby the approximate age at which menopause will occur.

(D) Terminologies in relation to menopause:

- **Natural Menopause:**
  It is recognised to have occurred after 12 months of amenorrhoea for which there are no obvious pathological causes.

- **Premenopause:**
  It is often used to refer to the entire reproductive period up to the final menstrual period (FMP).

- **Perimenopause**:
  It is the period immediately before 2 - 3 years and 1 year after FMP. It may last up to 3 - 5 yrs. The characteristics are:
  - Increasing serum FSH levels
  - Significantly reduced fertility
  - Erratic menstrual periods
  - Onset of menstrual symptoms
    (The term is used interchangeably with menopause transition.)

- **Climacteric:**
  It is interchangeably used with perimenopause and menopause transition. When associated with symptoms, it is called climacteric syndrome.
- **Postmenopause:**
  It is the span of life dating from the final

menstrual period onwards regardless of whether the menopause was spontaneous or iatrogenic.

- **Premature Ovarian Insufficiency (POI):** Premature Ovarian Insufficiency has replaced the term premature menopause. POI is described as amenorrhoea due to loss of ovarian function before the age of 40 years. It is a state of female hypergonadotropic hypogonadism. Its incidence is 1%. It can manifest as primary amenorrhoea with onset before menarche or secondary amenorrhoea with onset after the establishment of natural menses. Criteria for diagnosis of POI as per **European Society of Human Reproduction and Embryology (ESHRE 2015)** is **'Elevated FSH levels > 25 IU/L on two occasions > 4 weeks apart'**.

- **Early Menopause**: It is the time span between the spontaneous or iatrogenic menopause occurring between 40 years of age and the accepted typical age of menopause for a given population (between 40 and 46.2 years in Indian population). Incidence is 5%.

- **Delayed Menopause:** It is not well defined but may be important in terms of increased problems associated with hyperestrogenism. It is two SDs above from the natural average age of menopause in a given population. In India, we may consider it to be 54 years or more.

- **Postmenopausal Bleeding (PMB):** It is the bleeding which occurs 12 months after the last menstrual period. However, it is recommended that any vaginal bleeding that occurs 6 months after the last menstrual period should be investigated.

- **Induced Menopause/Surgical Menopause**:
  It is the cessation of menses due to bilateral oophorectomy or iatrogenic ablation of ovarian function or hysterectomy.

(E) Symptoms of Menopause:

- About 20% of women have no symptoms at all, while 60% have mild to moderate symptoms. The remaining 20% have severe symptoms that interfere with their daily life.

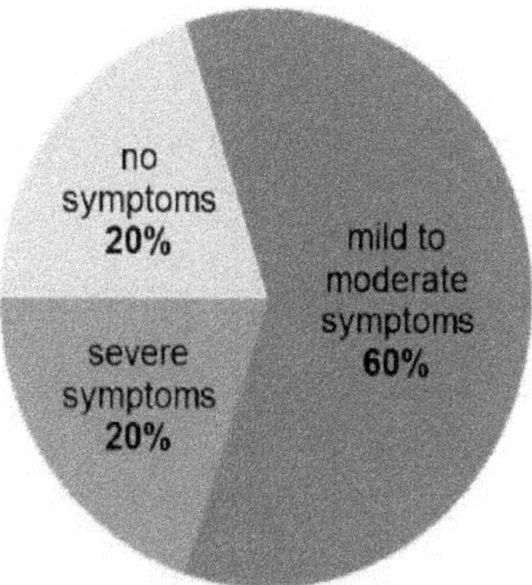

- Menopausal symptoms can be influenced by different factors, for example, your stage of life and general health and wellbeing.

- The biology and symptomatology of menopause is blurred due to its relationship to the underlying aging process.

- Vasomotor, urogenital symptoms and irregular menstrual periods are typically linked with serum oestrogen levels.

- Long term effects on bone and heart have been related to oestrogen deficiency.

- Many other symptoms like muscle and joint pain, vertigo, mood changes, depression, insomnia, nervousness have been associated with menopause but are not necessarily due to decrease in oestrogen levels.

- Many symptoms start during perimenopause and can continue into postmenopause. Australian studies show that some women experience symptoms like hot flashes and night sweats well into their 60s.

Physical Symptoms:

Physical symptoms may include:

- Irregular periods
- Hot flashes
- Night sweats
- Sleep problems
- Sore breasts
- Itchy, crawly or dry skin
- Exhaustion and fatigue
- Dry vagina
- Loss of sex drive (libido)
- Headaches or migraine
- Aches and pains
- Bloating
- Urinary problems

- Weight gain due to androgen-oestrogen ratio shift and low BMR.

Emotional symptoms:

Emotional symptoms may include:

- Feeling irritable or frustrated
- Feeling anxious
- Difficulty in concentrating
- Forgetfulness
- Mood swings

Symptoms and Disorders in Relation to Age and Menopause:

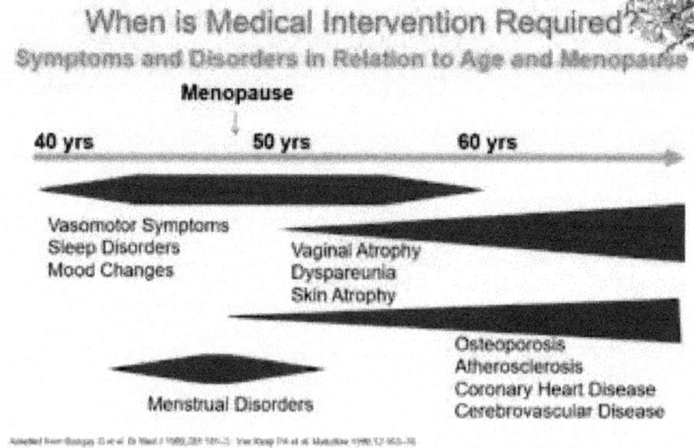

Source: Bungay G, et al. Br Med J 1980; 281: 181 - 3;

Van Keep PA, et al. Maturities 1990; 12:163-70.

- **The immediate symptoms of menopause transition are irregular periods, hot flashes, night sweats, sleep and mood disturbances, joint and muscle pain, vaginal dryness and low sexual desire**

which generally resolve over a while in mild cases.

- **Genitourinary symptoms appear in the early postmenopausal period and may worsen over some time if not treated.**

- **The long term consequences of menopause affect bone and cardiovascular health which worsen with aging.**

In next chapter, we will navigate the risk factors of cardiovascular disease in postmenopausal women.

CHAPTER III: UNRAVELING THE RISK FACTORS FOR CARDIOVASCULAR DISEASE

"Postmenopausal women have the power to rewrite their heart health story.

By prioritizing lifestyle changes and seeking appropriate medical care they can reclaim their vitality and reduce their risk of cardiovascular disease."

- Dr. John Smith

(A) Key Points:

- Cardiovascular disease (CVD) is the leading cause of death in United States and worldwide.

- Cardiovascular disease is number one killer in postmenopausal women, cancer being second.

- Women can develop heart disease at any age, but the risk increases after menopause, usually after the age of 55 years.

- It is assumed that estrogen is cardio protective in premenopausal women.

- Epidemiological evidence has shown that menopausal transition is associated with a higher prevalence of CVD risk factors such as central obesity, atherogenic dyslipidemia, insulin resistance and arterial hypertension.

- Menopause is often a turning point for women's health worldwide. Cardio metabolic changes can manifest at the menopause transition, superimposing the effect of ageing onto the risk of cardiovascular disease.

- **Menopause can be considered as a "Biological Marker of cardiovascular disease".**

- While average age for heart attack is 64.5 years for men and 70.3 years for women, nearly 20% of those who die of heart disease are under the age of 65 years.

- Cardiovascular diseases which are the leading cause of death in postmenopausal women include:
    - Coronary heart disease or Ischemic heart disease or Atherosclerotic heart disease or Atherosclerotic cardiovascular disease
    - Stroke and
    - Venous thromboembolism

- Coronary artery disease is the most common type of heart disease and the cause of heart attacks in women.

- Studies strongly suggest that there is association of increase in cardiovascular events after menopause, distinct from other risk factors common to both genders.

- Additionally, there are some nontraditional women-specific risk factors such as pregnancy complications, PCOD, autoimmune diseases and age at menarche.

(B) Gender Differences:

(Why women are at greater risk for CVD?)

- Prevalence of cardiovascular disease can vary between males and females and may be influenced by age. Generally men have a higher incidence of CVD in younger ages compared with women. This is partly attributed to the cardioprotective effects of estrogen in premenopausal women. However after menopause, the risk of CVD in women increases and eventually catches upto that of men.

- It is important to acknowledge that historically, CVD research has predominantly focused on men. This has led to a knowledge gap in understanding the unique aspects of CVD in women. As a result, symptoms and risk factors specific to women may be underdiagnosed and undertreated. It's taken more than a decade for doctors to realize that more women are affected due to CVD events in postmenopausal women.

- With men, heart disease typically manifests itself through the classic symptoms such as crushing or squeezing chest pain or tightness in the chest. Women on the other hand may occasionally present as chest pain but most often present with shortness of breath, pain in neck, jaw, throat, and upper abdomen or back. Women tends to have a lot of vague symptoms such as just being tired, not being able to say what's wrong with them. On the top of that 64% of women who die suddenly of coronary heart disease have no previous symptoms. And that's why succumb to death due to CVD without being treated in time.

- Women have smaller arteries than men, so coronary artery disease develop differently and more diffusely. Also CVD in women tends to affect micro branches of coronaries resulting in microvascular dysfunction. An angiogram, a procedure commonly preferred to look for the blockage may not always catch the disease, making treatment more challenging.

- Studies have shown that endogenous estrogen during reproductive period delays manifestation of atherosclerotic disease in women. And that may be the reason that CVD develops 7 – 10 years later in women than men and still the number one cause of death in women after the age of 65 years.

- WISE Study (Women's Ischemic Syndrome Evaluation Study), shows that young women with premature ovarian insufficiency (POI) have 7 fold increase in coronary artery disease risk. Again they have approximately 2 years lower life expectancy compared with women with a normal menopause.

- Obesity, another traditional risk factor is more prevalent in women than in men. Obesity has independently shown to be associated with increased risk of CVD.
    - According to the National Health and Nursing Examination Survey (NHNES) in 2013, among 37.7% of adults aged 20 years or older who are classified as obese, 40.4% were women as against 35% men.

    - Framingham Heart Study found obesity to increase relative risk of CVD by 64% in women compared with 46% in men.

    - Central obesity with an increase in visceral fat occurs more frequently after menopause in women, with a higher risk of comorbid risk factors and components of metabolic syndrome in women compared with ageing men.

- The risk of diabetes on CVD is different in women than in men. Diabetic women are disproportionately affected.

  - Mortality for diabetic women is an estimated 2.1 million versus 1.8 million in diabetic men, and majority of these deaths are cardiovascular in nature.

  - In women with DM, there is a 1.81 fold increased risk of death from ischemic heart disease compared with women without DM, while diabetic men has 1.48 fold increased risk when compared with nondiabetic men.

  - Risk of heart failure is 5 fold higher in diabetic women as compared with nondiabetic, while in diabetic men the risk is 2 fold as against nondiabetic men.

- Hypertension is another well-established risk factor for CVD and the leading cause of cardiovascular mortality worldwide. Women with hypertension have a higher population-adjusted cardiovascular mortality when compared with men and are less likely to be treated by guideline-directed blood pressure goals.

- At younger ages (< 50 years) smoking is more deleterious in women than in men, with a larger negative impact of the total number of cigarettes smoked per day. Smoking increases the risk of a first acute myocardial infarction relatively more in women than in men.

- Pregnancy complications such as pre-eclampsia, gestational diabetes and preterm births, autoimmune diseases, PCOD and age at menarche contribute additional risk factors in some women.

Heart disease used to be considered a man's disease, but no longer. While heart disease is on the decline among men, it is rising among women. Heart disease is number one killer in women over 35 worldwide accounting for more deaths every year than all cancers combined.

Source: Canadian Women's Heart Health Centre.

(C) Traditional Risk Factors for CVD applicable to both genders:

The genesis of cardiovascular disease is multifactorial. The factors contributing to the development of CVD starts at the intrauterine stage, which is called the '**Barkers Hypothesis.**' The other factors are:

1. Age
2. Family History
3. High Blood Pressure
4. High Cholesterol Levels
5. Uncontrolled Diabetes
6. Obesity
7. Smoking
8. Sedentary Lifestyle
9. Unhealthy Diet
10. Chronic Stress

It is important to note that these factors can interact with each other and with an individual's genetic predisposition, making it crucial to address and manage them to reduce the risk of cardiovascular disease.

Regular check-ups with healthcare professionals can help identify and manage these risk factors effectively.

In this book we are not going to discuss the traditional risk factors in detail common to both genders as mentioned above. **But here, we are interested more in women- specific risk factors which are contributing to CVD risk in women in addition to traditional risk factors common to both genders.**

(D) Women-Specific Risk Factors for CVD

Gender differences in pathophysiology, prevalence and impact of cardiovascular disease risk factors may explain the high cardiovascular mortality rates in women**. For better understanding women-specific risk factors can be described under 3 headings:**

1. **Estrogen as cardioprotective in premenopausal women.**
2. **Menopause as a risk factor of CVD due to estrogen deficiency.**
3. **Non-traditional risk factors in some women.**

Estrogen as cardioprotective in premenopausal women:

Estrogen has regulatory effect on several metabolic factors such as inflammatory markers, lipids and coagulatory system.

Cardioprotective effect of estrogen through its anti-inflammatory action:

- Estrogen has been found to exhibit anti-inflammatory properties, which can contribute to its cardioprotective effects in the prevention of CVD. Inflammation plays a significant role in the development and progression of cardiovascular disease including atherosclerosis.

- Estrogen has been shown to modulate the immune response and reduce the production of pro-inflammatory molecules in the body. It can inhibit the expression of certain inflammatory markers such as cytokines and adhesion molecules, which are involved in the initiation and progression of inflammation.

- By reducing inflammation, estrogen helps to maintain the integrity of blood vessels and prevent the formation of atherosclerotic plaques. Atherosclerosis is a condition characterized by the accumulation of cholesterol and immune cells in the arterial walls, leading to the narrowing and hardening of blood vessels. Estrogen's anti-inflammatory action can help inhibit the inflammatory process that contribute to the development of atherosclerosis.

- Additionally, estrogen has been shown to promote the production of anti-inflammatory molecules such as interleukin-10 (IL-10), which further helps to counteract inflammation and protect against CVD.

Cardioprotective effect of estrogen through its regulation on lipid profile:

- Estrogen plays a role in regulating lipid profile, specifically by influencing the role of different lipids in the blood stream. It has both direct and indirect effects on lipid metabolism.

- One way estrogen affects lipid profile is by increasing the levels of high density lipoprotein (HDL-C), often referred to as good cholesterol. HDL-C helps remove LDL-C, often referred as bad cholesterol from blood stream, reducing the risk of plaque buildup in the arteries.

- Estrogen also has indirect effects on lipid metabolism by influencing the activity of enzymes involved in lipid synthesis and breakdown. It can decrease the production of triglycerides, a type of fat found in blood, by inhibiting the enzyme lipoprotein lipase.

- Estrogen promotes and maintains gynecoid body fat distribution.

- Additionally, estrogen can increase the breakdown of LDL-C receptors, which help remove LDL-C from blood stream.

Cardioprotective effect of estrogen through its role in regulating the coagulatory system:

- Estrogen plays a role in regulating the coagulatory system, which is responsible for maintaining the balance between blood clotting and preventing the coagulatory system through various mechanisms.

- One way, estrogen influences the coagulatory system, is by increasing the production of certain clotting factors, such as fibrinogen and Van Willebrand factor. These clotting factors are essential for the formation of clots. Estrogen can also enhance the activity of other clotting factors such as factor VII, VIII and X.

- Additionally, estrogen has been found to decrease the production of certain anticoagulant proteins such as protein S and antithrombin III.

Cardioprotective effect of estrogen through Nitric Oxide (NO):

- Estrogen has been found to have a cardioprotective effect through its interaction with nitric oxide. Nitric Oxide plays crucial role in maintaining cardioprotective health. It helps to relax and dilate blood vessels, improving blood flow and reducing the risk of high blood pressure and subsequent CVD.

- Estrogen enhances the production and availability of nitric oxide by stimulating the production of endothelial nitric oxide synthase (eNOS), an enzyme responsible for synthesizing NO in endothelial cells lining the blood vessels. This increased production of nitric oxide helps to maintain the flexibility and health of blood vessels, preventing the development of atherosclerosis and reducing the risk of CVD.

Cardioprotective action of estrogen through its antioxidant effect:

- Antioxidants are substances that help neutralize harmful free radicals in the body, which can cause oxidative stress and damage cells, including those of cardiovascular system.

- Estrogen acts as an antioxidant by directly scavenging free radicals and inhibiting their harmful effects. It can donate an electron to stabilize the free radicals and prevent them in causing damage to cells and tissues. This antioxidant activity helps to reduce oxidative stress and protect CVS from damage.

- Estrogen also stimulates the production of endogenous antioxidants, such as **superoxide dismutase (SOD) and glutathione,** which further enhances its cardioprotective effect. These antioxidants help to neutralize free radicals and maintain the balance between oxidative stress and antioxidant defence in the body.

It is important to note that the mechanisms by which endogenous estrogen is cardioprotective in premenopausal women are complex and not fully understood. Researchers continue to study and explore the various ways in which estrogen protects blood vessels and cardiovascular system as a whole in premenopausal women.

Pathophysiology of CVD in postmenopausal women due to estrogen deficiency.

Estrogen deficiency in postmenopausal women can increase CVD risk through various mechanisms.

Endothelial Dysfunction:

- Estrogen deficiency can lead to impaired endothelial function, promoting the development of arterial stiffness and hypertension.

- Menopause has shown to be associated with more atherogenic shift in the lipid profile. Estrogen deficiency may result in unfavorable lipid changes disturbing the normal lipid profile, thus increasing the risk of atherosclerosis.

Menopause related lipid changes are:

- Increased total cholesterol (> 200 mg/dl)
- Increased triglycerides (> 150 mg/dl)
- Increased LDL-C (Bad cholesterol > 100 mg/dl)
- Increased lipoprotein (a)
- Decreased HDL-C (Good Cholesterol < 40 mg/dl)

Vasocontraction:

- Estrogen deficiency can lead to reduced Nitric Oxide (NO) formation resulting in narrowing of blood vessels which promotes further elevating blood pressure.

Abdominal or visceral obesity:

- After menopause, there is decrease in estrogen levels, which can lead to a shift in fat distribution. Fat tends to be redistributed from peripheral areas (such as hip and thigh) to the abdominal region. This central or visceral fat is more metabolically active and is associated with a higher risk of various health issues, including cardiovascular disease, type 2 diabetes and metabolic syndrome.

- Visceral fat is different from subcutaneous fat because it surrounds internal organs like liver, pancreas and intestines. It can release inflammatory substances and hormones that affect insulin resistance and overall metabolic health.

Main factors contributing to menopausal changes in body composition

Genetic factors	Hormonal factors	Exogenous factors
Genetic predisposition Ethnicity Epigenetic changes	Rapid hypoestrogenemia Relative hyperandrogenemia Low SHBG levels	Unhealthy nutrition Low physical activity Drugs (e.g. steroids, insulin) Diseases

Increase in body weight
Increase and redistribution of fat mass (from gynoid to abdominal obesity)
Decrease in fat-free mass

Metabolic Syndrome:

- Metabolic syndrome is a cluster of conditions that occurs together, increasing the risk of CVD and type 2 diabetes. To diagnose metabolic syndrome, a woman must have at least 3 of the following risk factors.

    - **Central Obesity**
      As per **WHO** criteria waist circumference >80 cm and waist-to-hip ratio > 0.85

    - **High Blood Pressure**
      Elevated blood pressure typically defined as 130/85 mm of Hg and more.

    - **Insulin Resistance**
      Elevated fasting blood sugar levels > 100 mg/dl or more, indicating insulin resistance or prediabetes or frank type 2 diabetes.

- **High triglycerides**
  >150 mg /dl

- **Low HDL-C**
  <40 mg /dl

- Each component of metabolic syndrome such as hypertension, dyslipidemia and insulin resistance can independently contribute to the development of CVD.

- The risk factors of metabolic syndrome can interact with each other, further increasing the risk of CVD. For example, insulin resistance can contribute to type 2 DM, hypertension and dyslipidemia, accelerating the development of atherosclerosis and ultimately CVD.

- Metabolic syndrome is associated with chronic low grade inflammation and increased oxidative stress, which can damage blood vessels and promote atherosclerosis.

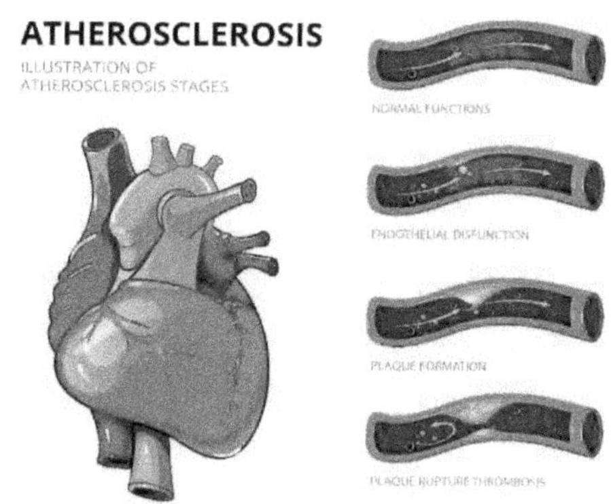

Fat that surrounds the heart is associated with increased risk of CVD.

- Postmenopausal women are at greater risk for heart disease due to a greater volume of a type of fat that surround the heart. Two types of fat that surrounds the heart are epicardial fat and Paracardial fat. Epicardial fat covers the heart tissue and is located between the outside of heart and the pericardium (a membrane that encases the heart). Epicardial fat is the energy source for the heart. While Paracardial fat, found outside the pericardium, there is no protective function of this fat. In fact the literature review showed that:

    - The greater Paracardial fat volume in postmenopausal women was not only linked to lower levels of estradiol, but it is also associated with a greater risk of coronary artery calcification, which is an early sign of heart disease.

    - Among the study participants, 60% increase in Paracardial fat was associated with a 45% increase in risk of coronary artery calcification in postmenopausal women compared with premenopausal women.

Prothrombotic State:

- Metabolic syndrome is linked to Prothrombotic state, meaning higher tendency for blood clot formation which can lead to heart attacks and strokes.

Overall, estrogen deficiency in postmenopausal women can contribute to an increased risk of developing CVD.

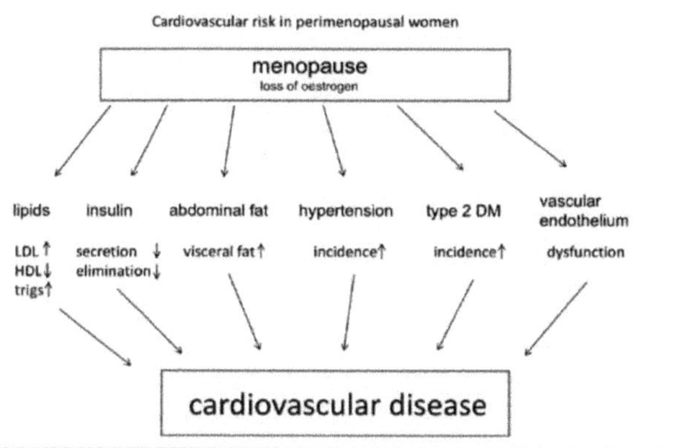

Non-traditional Risk Factors contributing to CVD in some women:

Apart from the traditional risk factors common to both genders and the menopause related risk factors, there are some additional nontraditional risk factors in some women, thereby increasing the risk of CVD.

Following are some of the Non-traditional Risk Factors. We will navigate them one by one.

1. **Pregnancy complications such as:**
    - Pre-eclampsia/Gestational Hypertension
    - Gestational Diabetes
    - Preterm Pregnancy
    - Multiple Pregnancy Losses

2. **Age at Menarche**

3. **PCOD (Polycystic Ovarian Disease)**

4. **Autoimmune Diseases**

Pregnancy Complications:

- Researchers have shown that women with history of adverse pregnancy outcomes are at increased risk of cardiovascular disease later in life.

- Pregnancy itself is considered to be the challenge to the maternal cardiovascular system. The maternal cardiovascular system goes through several important adaptations during pregnancy. The cardiac output, heart rate and stroke volume increases during pregnancy due to plasma volume expansion and systemic vascular dilatation. These changes may be attributed to the normal pregnancy outcomes in relation to growing fetus and the mother. Majority of the women withstand this **"Physiological Stress"** without any complications.

- In some women, who experience complications, either there is lack of development of above mentioned physiological changes in relation to cardiovascular disease or they cannot withstand these physiological stress resulting in pregnancy complications. Exact reason is not known as pregnancy complications are again multifactorial. Further research will clarify the things.

- Therefore, it may be assumed that pregnancy may be considered as a **"Physiological Stress Test"**, as the stress it places on woman's body may reveal underlying predisposition to CVD later in life that would otherwise remain hidden for many years as per some of the studies.

- ***Care guidelines from the American Heart Association and American College of***

Obstetrician & Gynecologist *encourage healthcare providers to ask about a women's pregnancy history and to consider above mentioned pregnancy complications for future heart disease.* ***American College of Obstetricians and gynecologist's guidelines recommend a yearly assessment to check blood pressure, cholesterol, weight and blood sugar levels for women with a history of early onset or recurrent pre-eclampsia.***

Link between pre-eclampsia and the risk of CVD later in life.

Pre-eclampsia is a relatively common complication of pregnancy with prevalence of 3 – 7%. It is the leading cause of morbidity and mortality for a pregnant woman and also has a significant burden on the healthcare system worldwide.

A 2017 systemic review and meta-analysis of 22 studies found that pre-eclampsia is associated with 4 fold increase in future heart failure risk and 2 fold increase in coronary heart disease, stroke and cardiovascular death.

Research studies have found that women who experience gestational hypertension/pre-eclampsia during pregnancy may be at higher risk of developing CVD later in life. The exact reasons for this association are not fully understood, but several factors are believed to play a role. Here are some of the risk factors.

- **Endothelial Dysfunction:**
  Gestational hypertension and pre-eclampsia can cause damage to the lining of blood vessels

(endothelium), leading to the impaired vascular function and increasing the risk of atherosclerosis.

- **Chronic Inflammation:**
  Both conditions involve inflammation and oxidative stress, which can contribute to the development of CVD events over time.

- **Insulin Resistance:**
  Gestational hypertension/pre-eclampsia have been linked to insulin resistance, which is a risk factor for type 2 DM and metabolic syndrome further increasing the risk of CVD.

- **Persistent hypertension (Chronic hypertension):**
  Women who experience gestational hypertension may have a higher likelihood of developing chronic hypertension after giving birth, which is significant risk factor for heart disease.

Link between gestational diabetes and the risk of CVD later in life

Here are some of the risk factors which contribute to increased CVD risk.

GDM affects 4-7 % of pregnancies.

20-60 % of women will develop type 2 DM later in life within 5-10 years of index pregnancy.

GDM is associated with 2 fold risk of future cardiovascular events, with the risk being apparent within 10 years after pregnancy.

Here are some of the key factors:

- **Insulin Resistance:**
  Gestational diabetes is characterized by insulin resistance, where the body cells do not respond effectively to insulin. The condition may persist after pregnancy and can lead to the development of type 2 DM, which is a significant risk factor for CVD.

- **Atherosclerosis:**
  Insulin resistance and chronically high blood sugar levels can promote the development of atherosclerosis.

Link between preterm delivery and risk of CVD later in life

Preterm delivery refers to giving birth before 37 weeks of gestation and is associated with certain maternal health implications including the risk of CVD.

According to the statistics available from CDC (Centre for Disease Control and Prevention), premature birth affects approximately 1 in 10 babies in United States.

Researchers analyzed existing data on 70182 women from the **Nurses Health Study-2**: one of the largest ongoing studies into the risk factors for major chronic diseases in women. The study revealed that preterm delivery correlated with a 40 % higher risk of developing CVD compared with women who gave birth at term. The risk increased for women who had more than one preterm delivery. Women who delivered earlier than 32 weeks had double the risk of developing CVD.

According to the American Heart Association (AHA), women already have a risk of dying from CVD of 33 %. This number rises to 36 % for those who give birth 3-7 weeks before term and rises as 60 % for women who deliver 8 weeks or more prematurely.

Several factors contribute to this association:

- **Inflammation and oxidative stress:** Preterm delivery can cause stress on the maternal cardiovascular system, leading to increased inflammation and oxidative stress which are known risk factors for CVD.

- **Association with pre-eclampsia:** Sometimes pregnancy is terminated prematurely for uncontrolled severe pre-eclampsia. Pre-eclampsia itself is linked to increased risk of CVD.

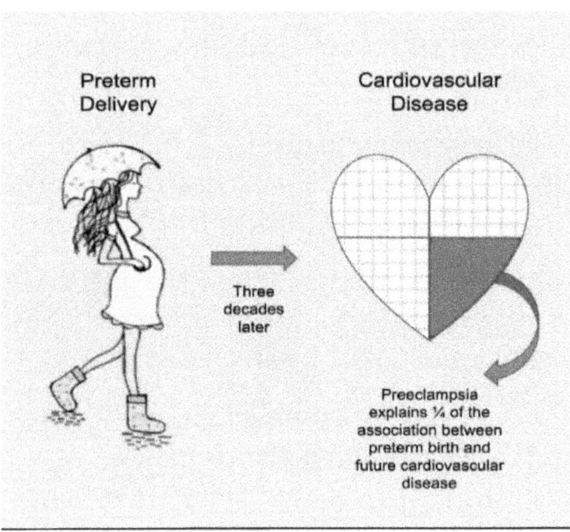

Link between multiple pregnancy losses and the risk of CVD later in life

Research has shown that there might be a link between multiple pregnancy losses (Recurrent miscarriages and stillbirths) and the risk of CVD later in life for women. The potential mechanisms linking multiple pregnancy losses and CVD are not fully understood, but several factors do play a role.

- **Chronic Stress:**
  Going through multiple pregnancy losses can lead to chronic stress which may contribute to inflammation and negatively affect cardiovascular health.

- **Immune System Dysregulation:**
  Multiple pregnancy losses may trigger immune system, potentially leading to inflammation and other CVD risk factors.

- **Shared Risk Factors:**
  Women who experience multiple pregnancy losses may have other underlying health conditions like hypertension, diabetes or risk factors that can also increase their CVD risk.

Link between age at menarche and the risk of CVD later in life

Menarche, a first menstruation, is the milestone event of pubertal development in girls since it represents the onset of female reproductive capacity.

Menarche is a complex phenomenon that is influenced by genetic and environmental factors.

According to the recent review, the age at menarche has remained stable between 12-16 years over the past few decades.

Age at menarche has been studied in relation to CVD risk later in life. Several research studies have explored this association. The exact mechanism behind this association is not fully understood, but it is believed that hormonal and metabolic changes during puberty may influence CVD health later in life.

In Korean population, menarche before 12 years (precocious menarche) has been linked to increased prevalence of obesity, insulin resistance and dyslipidemia in adulthood, culminating in higher CVD risk.

In a large population-based study in China, it has been found that those who had late menopause (after 15 years) had a higher risk of obesity, hypertension, diabetes and CVD risk compared with other women.

Link between PCOS (Polycystic Ovarian Syndrome) and risk of CVD later in life.

Polycystic Ovarian Syndrome is a disease that affects the endocrine, metabolic and reproductive systems and manifest in the reproductive age group.

The global prevalence of PCOS is estimated between 4% and 20%. The World Health Organization **(WHO)** data suggests that approximately 116 million women are affected by PCOS globally.

Common clinical presentations of PCOS include:

- **Irregular or infrequent menstrual cycles**
  Women with PCOS often experience irregular and infrequent menstrual cycles, which can lead to difficulty in predicting the ovulation resulting difficulty in conceiving and present in the clinics to seek advice for conception.

- **Weight Gain**
  Many women with PCOS find it difficult to lose weight, especially around abdomen.

- **Excessive hair growth**
  Increased levels of androgens in PCOS can lead to hirsutism (excessive hair growth on face, chest, back etc.)

- **Acne and oily skin**
  Elevated androgens can also contribute to the development of acne and oily skin.

Several Factors contribute PCOS association with CVD later in life:

Insulin Resistance:

Many women with PCOS have insulin resistance, a condition where the body cells do not respond effectively to insulin. Insulin resistance can lead to higher levels of insulin and glucose in the blood stream, increasing the risk of type 2 diabetes and metabolic syndrome. Both these conditions are risk factors for CVD.

Obesity:

PCOS is often linked with obesity, and excess weight can contribute to insulin resistance, inflammation and other factors that raise the risk of CVD.

Dyslipidemia:

PCOS can lead to changes in lipid profile, including elevated levels of LDL-C and triglycerides; and reduced levels of HDL-C. Imbalances in lipid levels are associated with an increased risk of CVD.

Inflammation:

PCOS is associated with chronic low grade inflammation in the body. Inflammation plays a role in the development of atherosclerosis and increases the risk of CVD.

Androgen levels:

Elevated levels of androgen in PCOS can contribute to insulin resistance, dyslipidemia and inflammation, all of which are risk factors for CVD.

Endothelial Dysfunction:

PCOS may lead to endothelial dysfunction. Endothelial dysfunction is early marker of cardiovascular disease.

Link between autoimmune diseases and CVD later in life

Autoimmune diseases are conditions in which the body's immune system mistakenly attacks healthy cells, tissues and organs leading to inflammation and damage. There are numerous type of autoimmune diseases including rheumatoid arthritis, systemic lupus erythematosus (SLE), multiple sclerosis, psoriasis etc.

80 % of all individuals affected by autoimmune diseases tend to be women due to variation within the sex chromosomes (XX) and hormonal changes.

- **Every 10 patients diagnosed with SLE, 9 are women.**
- **Out of every 7 patients diagnosed of rheumatoid arthritis, 5 are women.**

- **Systemic Sclerosis is 4 times more likely to occur in women.**

An International Research Team led by KU Leuven published the results of an epidemiological investigation into possible links between 19 of the most common autoimmune diseases and CVD. The results showed that patients with autoimmune disorder have a substantial higher risk **(between 1.4 to 3.6 times)** of developing CVD than people without autoimmune disorder.

Factors contributing the risks for developing CVD.

- The connection between autoimmune disease and the risk of CVD is postmenopausal women is primarily due to chronic inflammation. When the immune system remains in a state of constant activation, it releases inflammatory molecules that can damage blood vessels and promote the development of atherosclerosis.

- Atherosclerosis can lead to the formation of plaques within the arterial walls, which restrict blood flow to the heart causing heart attack or brain causing stroke; it can be life-threatening.

- Postmenopausal women are already at an increased risk of CVD due to hormonal changes associated with menopause. When risk due to autoimmune disease is added to the mix, the risk is further amplified.

(E) Work-up to identify risk factors for CVD at menopause clinic

The aim of establishing menopausal clinics is to screen and diagnose specific menopause-related problems and to assess the general condition of a woman by history, clinical examination and basic laboratory tests and plan for individualized management strategies.

The menopause transition or perimenopause is the **"Window of Opportunity"** to screen and to treat women for non-communicable diseases.

The concept of menopausal health is about women getting and staying healthy throughout life and should celebrate postmenopausal life with strength, energy and certain goals.

The Centre for Disease Control and Prevention urges all women to make healthy living a priority.

At menopause clinic primary healthcare provider is a gynecologist who takes detailed history, does physical examination including pelvic and breast examination, investigates her, identifies risk factors and formulate a plan for individualized counseling and treatment. The approach is basically multi-speciality oriented and the patients are **referred to respective speciality for proper treatment.**

Here we will only discuss the points which are in relation with assessing **the potential risk factors in causation of cardiovascular events in future in postmenopausal women.**

History taking for finding out risk factor for CVD:

Personal medical history:

- Hypertension

- Hyperlipidemia
- Diabetes
- Previous cardiovascular events if any
- Chronic kidney disease
- Autoimmune diseases like rheumatoid arthritis, SLE etc.
- Sleep apnea

Reproductive history:

- Age at menarche
- Polycystic Ovarian Syndrome (PCOS)
- Pregnancy complications if any
    - Gestational hypertension/Pre-eclampsia
    - Gestational diabetes
    - Preterm delivery
    - Multiple pregnancy losses
- Age at menopause

Lifestyle factors:

- Dietary habits
- Physical activity level
- Smoking
- Alcohol consumption

Present medication history:

- Use of blood pressure medications
- Use of cholesterol lowering medications
- Medications for diabetes
- Any other medications like steroids

Psychological factors:

- Chronic stress
- Anxiety and depression

Family medical history:

- Cardiovascular diseases (e.g. heart attack, stroke) in parents, siblings and close relatives.
- Cardiovascular events earlier in life in family members.

Physical Examination:

Physical examination should focus on identifying signs and markers that could indicate increased risk of cardiovascular events. It should be comprehensive and tailored to the individual's medical history and risk factors. Here are some points to be included in physical examination.

Blood pressure measurement:

Obtain accurate blood pressure readings to assess for hypertension, a major risk factor for cardiovascular disease. (Normal Blood Pressure: 120/80 mm of Hg.)

Body Mass Index (BMI) Calculation:

Calculate BMI: weight in kg/ (height in meter) 2 to evaluate weight status and potential obesity-related risks. (Normal BMI: 18.5 – 24.9 kg/m2).

Waist Circumference:

Measure waist circumference and waist-to-hip to assess central adiposity (visceral adiposity), which is associated with increased CVD risk. (Normal waist circumference: <80 cms and waist-to-hip ratio < 0.85 as per WHO criteria.)

Palpation of peripheral pulses:

Check peripheral pulses (e.g. radial, femoral, pedal) to assess for peripheral arterial disease.

Auscultation of heart sounds:

Listen for abnormal heart sounds if any (murmur, extra heart sounds) that may indicate underlying heart conditions.

Assessment of Jugular Venous Pressure (JVP):

Examine JVP to assess for signs of heart failure or fluid overload.

Assessment of Thyroid gland:

Palpate thyroid gland for any abnormality that could contribute to cardiovascular risk.

Examination of lower extremities:

Look for signs for edema, varicose veins and skin changes that might indicate circulatory issues.

Skin examination:

Look for xanthomas (cholesterol deposits) and skin manifestations of lipid disorders.

Respiratory examination:

Assess for signs of lung congestion or respiratory issues that could affect cardiovascular health.

Fundoscopic examination by the ophthalmologist:

Evaluate the retina for signs of hypertensive retinopathy or other vascular changes.

Neurological examination:

Evaluate neurological status, including reflexes and sensations, which can provide insides into overall vascular health.

Investigations:

In the cardiovascular risk assessment for postmenopausal women, the choice of investigations may vary based on the individual's risk factors and clinical presentation. Choice of investigations should be tailored to each individual's risk factors, symptoms and medical history. Here are some investigations that may be advised.

Blood Tests:

Lipid Profile: Normal values:

- Total Cholesterol: < 200 mg/dl
- Triglycerides: < 150 mg/dl
- LDL-C: < 100 mg/dl
- HDL-C: > 40 mg/dl

Fasting Blood Sugar: Normal values: < 100 mg/dl

HbA1C: Monitors long-term glucose control**:** Normal values: Between 4 – 5.6 %. Levels between 5.7 and 6.4 suggest that you are prediabetes and a higher chance of getting diabetes.

High-Sensitive C - reactive protein (hs-CRP): Measures inflammation: Normal value: less than 0.3 mg/dl. Minor elevation (0.3-1 mg/dl) can be seen in obesity, diabetes, sedentary lifestyle, cigarette smoking, pregnancy and genetic polymorphism.

Homocysteine levels: Evaluate vascular health: Normal value: Most lab reports normal ranges of homocysteine as about 4 – 15 microml/L.

Thyroid function tests: Detects deranged functions in relation to thyroid gland.

Renal function tests (RFT): Detects deranged functions in relation to kidney.

Complete Blood Count (CBC): Detects anemia and other blood related issues.

Following investigations are not mandatory and should be advised judiciously by physician/cardiologist depending upon the risk factors and the presenting symptoms.

- Electrocardiogram
- Echocardiogram
- Stress Testing
- Coronary Calcium Scoring
- Carotid Ultrasound
- Cardiac Biomarkers
- Pulmonary Function Test and so on.

Women with abnormal parameters should be referred to physician/cardiologist for correction of the risk factors and also for further advice and follow-ups.

All women should be counseled for healthy lifestyle to have a vibrant life ahead.

(F) Lifestyle modifications to keep yourself away from heart attacks:

By adopting a healthy lifestyle, you can help keep your blood pressure, cholesterol, blood sugars and body weight within normal limits; and lower your risk of heart attacks.

Here are some lifestyle changes that postmenopausal women can adopt to help reduce the risk of cardiovascular disease.

Eat a heart-healthy diet: Focus on consuming a balanced diet rich in fruits, vegetables, whole grains, lean proteins and healthy fats. Limit the intake of saturated and trans fats, sodium and added sugars. Unhealthy fats like saturated and trans fats can raise cholesterol levels and increase the risk of heart disease. Too much sodium can contribute to high blood pressure, which is a risk factor for heart disease. Excessive sugar intake can contribute to weight gain and increase the risk of heart disease. Minimize consumption of desserts and processed snacks. Opt for natural sources of sweetness like fruits.

Maintain healthy weight: Aim for a healthy body weight by incorporating regular physical activity and mindful food choices. Losing excess weight, if necessary, can help reduce the risk of cardiovascular disease. Be mindful of portion sizes to avoid overeating. Use smaller plates and bowls and pay attention to hunger and fullness cues.

Stay physically active: Engage in regular physical activities such as brisk walking, swimming, cycling or dancing. Aim for at least 150 minutes of moderate-intensity or 75 minutes of vigorous-intensity aerobic activity per week along with strength training exercises.

Quit smoking: If you smoke, quitting is one of the most important steps you can take to improve heart health.

Manage Stress: Find healthy ways to manage stress, such as practicing relaxation techniques, engaging in hobbies, spending time with loved ones, or seek professional help if needed. Chronic stress can contribute to cardiovascular disease risk.

Control blood pressure and cholesterol levels: Regularly monitor and manage your blood pressure and cholesterol levels through lifestyle modifications and if necessary, with the medications prescribed by your healthcare provider.

Limit alcohol consumption: If you choose to drink alcohol, do so in moderation. This means up to one drink per day for women.

Stay hydrated: Drink plenty of water throughout the day to maintain proper hydration. Limit sugary cold drinks and excessive caffeine intake.

Get regular check-ups: Schedule regular check-ups with your healthcare provider to monitor your overall health, discuss any concerns and receive appropriate screenings and preventive care.

Heart-friendly Diet and Heart-friendly physical activities:

Although some factors like age and genetics are beyond our control, 80 % of the risk of cardiovascular disease can be prevented by healthy eating and regular physical activities.

People are relying on vitamins and minerals rather than diet, exercise and healthy lifestyle and that's probably not good.

Heart-friendly Diet:

A heart-friendly diet for postmenopausal women should focus on maintaining a healthy weight, managing cholesterol levels, thereby promoting overall health. Here are some of the dietary guidelines.

1. **Increase Fiber Intake**
   Increase whole grains, fruits, green vegetables, legumes and nuts in your diet. High fiber foods help lower cholesterol level and improve heart health.

2. **Choose Healthy Fats**
   Opt for sources of unsaturated fats like olive oil, avocados and nuts. Limit saturated and trans fats found in fried foods and processed snacks.

3. **Lean Proteins**
   Choose lean protein sources like fish, skinless poultry, beans and lentils. Fish rich in omega-3 fatty acids (such as salmon) can be particularly beneficial for heart.
4. **Reduce Sodium**
   Limit your sodium intake to help manage blood pressure. Avoid processed foods, canned soups and excess salts in cooking.
5. **Increase Omega-3 fatty acids**
   Consume sources of omega-3 fatty acids, such as fatty fish, flaxseeds, chia seeds and walnuts to reduce inflammation and support heart health.
6. **Limit added sugars**
   Minimize sugary foods and beverages as they can contribute to weight gain and increase the risk of heart disease.
7. **Control Portion Sizes**
   Be mindful of portion sizes to avoid overeating and manage weight effectively.
8. **Choose low-fat dairy**
   Opt for low fat or non-fat dairy products to reduce saturated fat intake.
9. **Colorful Variety**
   Consume a colorful array of fruits and vegetables to get a wide range of antioxidants, vitamins and minerals.
10. **Stay hydrated**
    Drink plenty of water throughout the day to support overall health.

Fiber-rich foods help lower cholesterol levels and improve heart health. Here are some excellent sources of dietary fiber.

1. **Legumes:**
   - Lentils
   - Chickpeas

- Black beans
- Kidney beans
- Pinto beans

2. **Whole Grains:**
    - Oats
    - Quinoa
    - Brown rice
    - Whole wheat pasta
    - Barley

3. **Fruits**
    - Apples (with skin)
    - Pears (with skin)
    - Berries (raspberries, blackberries, strawberries)
    - Oranges
    - Bananas

4. **Vegetables**
    - Broccoli
    - Brussels sprouts
    - Carrots
    - Spinach
    - Kale

5. **Nuts and Seeds:**
    - Almonds
    - Chia seeds
    - Flaxseeds
    - Sunflower seeds
    - Pistachios

6. **Whole Grain Cereals:**
    - Bran cereals (like bran flakes)
    - Whole grain oat cereals

7. **Whole Grain Bread:**
    - Look for bread labeled as "whole grain or whole wheat"

8. **Popcorn:**
    - Air-popped popcorn is a whole grain snack high in fiber. (with no butter)

9. **Dry Fruits:**
    - Prunes
    - Raisins
    - Dried apricots (consume in moderation due to natural sugars)

10. **Sweet Potatoes:**
    An excellent source of fiber and vitamins.

Inclusion of healthy sources of fats (unsaturated fats) in diet is important for overall health and wellbeing. Here are some examples of healthy fatty foods that you can incorporate in your meals.

1. **Avocado**
    Avocados are rich in monounsaturated fats, which are heart-friendly fats that can help improve cholesterol levels.

2. **Olive oil**
    Olive oil is a staple of Mediterranean diet and is high in monounsaturated fats. It is used for cooking and drizzling over salads.

3. **Nuts**
   Almonds, walnuts, pistachios and other nuts are sources of healthy fats, fiber and various nutrients.

4. **Seeds**
   Chia seeds, flaxseeds and pumpkin seeds are rich in omega-3 fatty acids and provide a boost of healthy fats, fiber and nutrients.

5. **Fatty fish**
   Salmon, mackerel, sardines and trout are excellent sources of omega-3 fatty acids, which have been shown to support heart and brain health.

6. **Coconut**
   Coconut oil and coconut products can be used in cooking and baking. Coconut contains medium-chain triglycerides that are metabolized differently by the body.

7. **Seaweed**
   Seaweed and algae-based products like spirulina are sources of healthy fats, minerals and antioxidants.

8. **Dark chocolates**
   Dark chocolate with high cocoa content (70 % or higher) contain healthy fats and antioxidants. Enjoy in moderation.

9. **Chia pudding**
   Chia seeds soaked in liquid (such as almond milk) create a pudding that's high in healthy fats and fiber.

10.Olives

Olives are rich in monounsaturated fats and can be added to salads, sandwiches and Mediterranean dishes.

Eating more saturated or unhealthy fats can raise your cholesterol levels and increase your risk of heart disease. Hence there should be restricted use of saturated fats in diet. Average woman should not eat more than 20 gms of saturated fats per day. Here are some examples of unhealthy or saturated fats containing food.

- **Butter, ghee, cheese**
- **Processed foods like biscuits, cakes, chips etc.**
- **Fatty cuts of meat**
- **Pastries such as pies, quiches, sausage rolls**
- **Cream, crème fraiche, sour cream**
- **Ice cream, milkshakes**

How to avoid trans fats?

Trans fats are the worst type of fats as they raise LDL-C and lowers HDL-C in our body. Trans fats have been linked to high blood pressure, diabetes, dyslipidemia, obesity and ultimately to heart disease.

- Avoid using "Vanaspati" ghee for any type of cooking.
- When deep frying foods like Puri, Pakoda, Samosa etc., do not heat the oil for longer time.
- Avoid leaving the food in the oil for a longer period.
- **Do not reheat the oil or reuse the same oil for frying.** The oil which has been once

used for frying, can be used for preparation of vegetables, dal etc.

Heart-friendly physical activities for prevention of cardiovascular events:

Engaging in regular physical activity is crucial for maintaining heart health. Here are some heart-friendly exercises. Healthcare provider may help you determine the appropriate level of exercise and may provide personalized recommendations based on your personal health need.

- **Aerobic Exercises:**
  Aim for at least 150 minutes of moderate-intensity aerobic exercise or 75 minutes of vigorous aerobic exercise per week. Activities can include brisk walking, jogging, swimming, cycling and dancing.

- **Walking:**
  Walking is a low impact exercise that can be easily incorporated into your daily routine. It helps improve cardiovascular fitness and supports weight management. **Walking is a wonderful drug. Walking for an average of 30 minutes or more can lower the risk of heart disease, stroke by 35% and type 2 diabetes by 40%.**

- **Swimming:**
  Swimming provides a full-body workout. It helps improve cardiovascular endurance, muscle strength and flexibility.

- **Cycling:**
  Cycling, whether outdoors or on a stationary bike, is a great way to improve heart health and leg strength. It's also a low-impact exercise.

- **Dancing:**
  Dance-based fitness classes or even dancing at home can be a fun and effective way to increase heart rate and improve cardiovascular fitness.

- **Strength Training:**
  Incorporate strength training exercises using light weights or resistance bands. Building muscle mass can help boost metabolism and improve overall health.

- **Yoga:**
  Yoga promotes flexibility, balance and relaxation.

- **Tai Chi:**
  This mind-body exercise combines slow, flowing movements with deep breathing. It helps improve balance, flexibility and relaxation.

- **Staying Active:**
  Engage in activities you enjoy, such as gardening, dancing around the house or playing with grandchildren. Every bit of movements adds up.

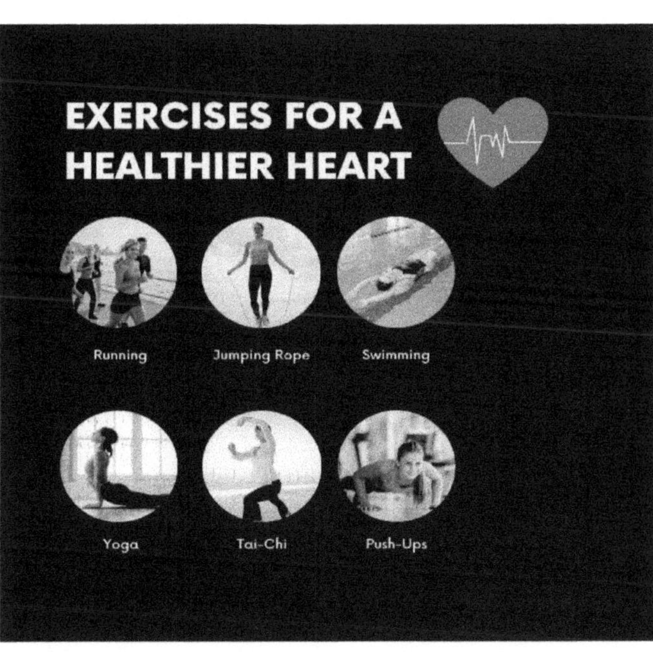
EXERCISES FOR A
HEALTHIER HEART
Running
Jumping Rope
Swimming
Yoga
Tai-Chi
Push-Ups

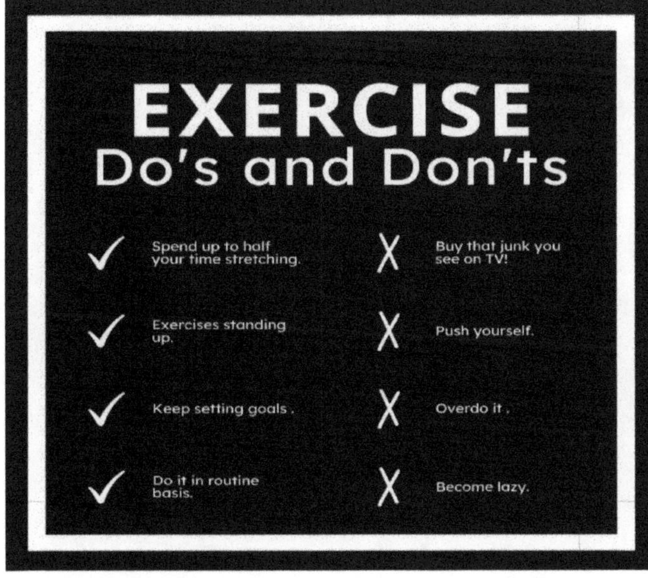
EXERCISE
Do's and Don'ts
Spend up to half your time stretching.
Buy that junk you see on TV!
Exercises standing up.
Push yourself.
Keep setting goals .
Overdo it .
Do it in routine basis.
Become lazy.

Why Aerobic exercises are considered as "Heart-Friendly"?

Aerobic exercises are considered heart-friendly because they provide a range of benefits that specifically target and improve cardiovascular health. It is important to start gradually and choose aerobic exercises that you enjoy and sustain. Do remember to warm up before exercising and cool down afterword to prevent injury. If you have any existing health conditions or concerns, it's a good idea to consult with a healthcare provider before beginning a new exercise. Here's why aerobic exercises are beneficial for your heart.

1. **Strengthens the heart:**
   During aerobic activities, heart pumps more blood to supply oxygen and nutrients to the muscles and organs. Over the time, this strengthens the heart muscle, making it more efficient at pumping blood and improving overall cardiac function.

2. **Improve Circulation:**
   Aerobic exercises help dilate blood vessels, which enhances blood flow through the body. This helps reduce the strain on blood vessels and lowers blood pressure, reducing risk of heart diseases.

3. **Increase in Cardiac Output:**
   Cardiac output is the amount of blood, heart pumps per minute. Aerobic exercises increase cardiac output by making the heart beat more efficiently and effectively, which can result in better circulation.

4. **Lower Cholesterol Levels:**
   Regular exercise can help raise levels of HDL-C, often referred to as good cholesterol and lower levels of LDL-C, known as bad cholesterol. This

contributes to a healthier lipid profile which is needed to keep cardiovascular system healthier.

5. **Weight Management:**
   Engaging in aerobic activities burns calories and helps with weight management. Maintaining a healthy weight reduces the risk of conditions like high blood pressure, diabetes and heart disease.

6. **Enhance Oxygen Utilization:**
   Aerobic exercises improve your body's ability to use oxygen efficiently.

7. **Reduce Inflammation:**
   Regular aerobic exercise can help reduce chronic inflammation, a factor that plays a role in the development of cardiovascular disease.

8. **Stress Reduction:**
   Aerobic activities stimulate the release of endorphins, which are natural mood lifters. Reduced stress contribute to better heart health.

9. **Better Blood Sugar Control:**
   Aerobic exercise improves insulin sensitivity, helping to regulate blood sugar levels. This particularly important for preventing or managing diabetes, which can impact heart health.

10. **Long-term Heart Health:**
    Engaging in consistent aerobic activities over time contributes in maintaining heart health and reducing the risk of cardiovascular events as heart attacks and strokes.

(G) Role of Menopause Hormone Therapy (MHT) in preventing CVD

Key Points:

- Initiation of MHT is a safe option for healthy asymptomatic women who are within 10 years of menopause or younger than 60 years of age and who do not have other contraindications to MHT.

- MHT is not to be used for primary or secondary prevention of cardiovascular disease.

- At any age, avoid MHT in women with high risk of CVD or with established CVD.

- MHT is effective in reducing vasomotor symptoms associated with perimenopause or menopause, promoting bone health and in many cases improving quality of life.

- A Cochrane review including 24 randomized controlled trials studying MHT administration for vasomotor symptoms demonstrated a reduction in weekly hot flashes by 75% and a 87% decrease in severity of hot flashes, demonstrating it **to be an effective therapy for this difficult-to-manage symptoms of menopause, which on its own is associated with increased risk of CVD.**

- MHT is cardioprotective, if started in perimenopause or early postmenopause for vasomotor symptoms in healthy women. It reduces the risk of type 2 diabetes and has positive effect on the lipid profile and metabolic syndrome.

- Randomized controlled data from a **Danish Osteoporosis Trials** have shown that MHT reduced the incidence of coronary heart disease by around 50% and reduced overall mortality if commenced within 10 years of menopause and below 60 years of age.

- **Early vs Late Intervention Trial with Estradiol (ELITE 2016)** reported that ET resulted in significantly lower risk of atherosclerosis progression when therapy initiated within 6 years of menopause. But this effect was not seen in the late postmenopausal women when therapy initiated 10 or more years after menopause.

- **The Kronos Early Estrogen Prevention Study (KEEPS)** evaluated the effectiveness of a combined estrogen/ progestin in preventing progression of carotid intima-media thickness (CIMT) or coronary artery calcium (CAC) in women who are within 36 months of their final menstrual period.

- **The SMART (Selective Estrogen Menopause and Response to Therapy)** trials have gone a step further in evaluating effects of conjugated estrogens/bazedoxifene (Bazedoxifene 20 mg/CEE 0.45 mg) on postmenopausal women. At 12 months, this combination was associated with significant improvements in total cholesterol, LDL-C and HDL-C levels when compared with placebo. (Triglyceride levels, however were significantly increased.)

CHAPTER IV: POSTMENOPAUSAL OSTEOPOROSIS

It is never too early to start

prevention of osteoporosis,

It is never too late to start

treatment of osteoporosis.

(A) Do postmenopausal women should take osteoporosis seriously?

- Osteoporosis is particularly dangerous in postmenopausal women because the hormonal changes that occur during menopause lead to a significant decrease in estrogen levels. Estrogen plays a crucial role in maintaining bone density and strength.

- Osteoporosis is not a terminal illness and does not itself directly influence life expectancy. However, having a fracture especially in spine and hip, which is obvious even with a lesser trauma (as the bones are fragile), can definitely prove fatal.

- **Studies have shown that, despite improvements in the treatment of hip fractures, only 60% recover all their previous functions. Between 7.9 – 26.9% die within 3 to 6 months and 25% have levels of disability that require constant care throughout life.**

(B) Osteoprotective role of estrogen in premenopausal women:

Estrogen plays a significant role in maintaining bone health through several mechanisms.

- **Bone Remodelling Regulation:**
  Estrogen helps regulate the balance between bone resorption (breakdown of old bone tissue) and bone formation (creation on new bone tissue). It inhibits the activity of osteoclasts, cells responsible for bone resorption, and promotes the activity of osteoblasts, cells responsible for bone formation. This balance ensures that the bone density is maintained.

- **Calcium Absorption:**
  Estrogen enhances the absorption of calcium from the intestine, which in an essential mineral for bone strength. Calcium is a key component of bone mineralization, and maintaining proper calcium levels in the body is crucial for preventing bone loss.

- **Inhibition of Apoptosis:**
  Estrogen prevents apoptosis (programmed cell death) of osteoblasts, the cells responsible for bone health. This ensures a continuous supply of new bone tissue.

- **Stimulation of Growth factors:**
  Estrogen stimulates the production of various growth factors that promote bone growth and healing.

- **Collagen Synthesis:**
  Estrogen contributes to the synthesis of collagen, a structural protein that provides flexibility and strength to bones.

- **Maintenance of Bone Blood Flow:**
  Estrogen helps maintain healthy blood flow to bones, ensuring that they receive the necessary nutrients and oxygen for optimal functioning.

- **During menopause, when estrogen levels decline, these protective mechanisms become compromised. The increased bone resorption and decreased bone formation contribute to the gradual loss of bone density and strength, leading to osteoporosis.**

(C) Understanding Osteoporosis:

Definition:

- The word osteoporosis is derived from Greek roots: **osteon** meaning bone and **poros** meaning little holes. Osteoporosis literally means porous bones, first described in 1894.

- World Health Organization (**WHO**) defines osteoporosis as a systemic skeletal disease characterized by:
  - Low bone mass,
  - with micro architectural deterioration of bone tissue,
  - with a consequent increase in bone fragility and susceptibility to fractures involving the wrist, spine, hip, pelvis, ribs or humerus.

- Osteoporosis is frequently called the "**Silent Killer**" because it itself has no symptoms. The patients are unaware of their bone loss until they experience a fracture. The disease can also affect the oral health when the density of bone around the tooth lessens, tooth can become loose.

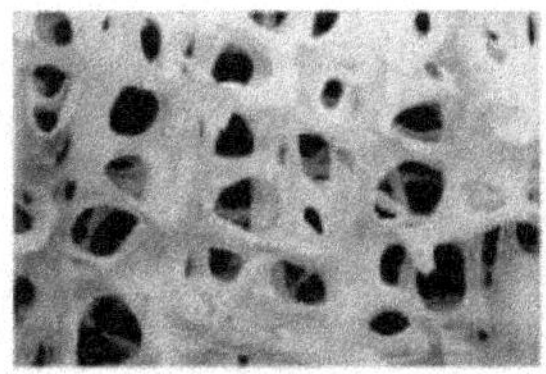

Normal Bone

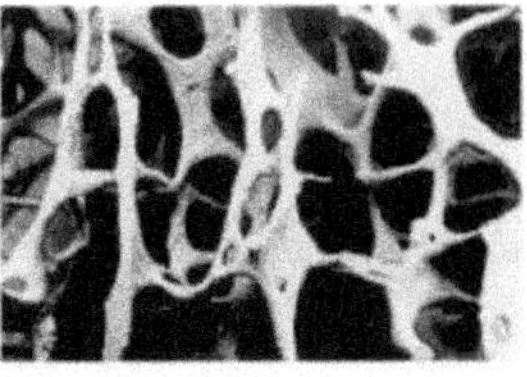

Osteoporotic bone

- As a consequence of increased life expectancy, osteoporosis is emerging as a major health problem in postmenopausal women and elderly men.

- Osteoporosis is underdiagnosed and undertreated despite the fact that prevention and treatment options are available.

- In severe cases, even mild to moderate trauma i.e. fall from sitting or standing position can caused fractures – fragility fractures.

- Patients with osteoporotic fractures suffer from high morbidity, increased risk of another fracture and a high risk of mortality. Overall hip fracture causes the most morbidity and mortality.

- Reported mortality rates in hip fractures are up to 20-24% in the first year.
- Loss of function with dependence among survivors is profound, with 40% unable to walk independently and 60% require assistance a year later.

(D) Prevalence, magnitude and burden of osteoporosis worldwide

- It is estimated that osteoporosis affects over 200 million women worldwide. $1/10^{th}$ of women aged 60, $1/5^{th}$ of women aged 70, $2/5^{th}$ of women aged 80 and $2/3^{rd}$ of women aged 90 carry this diagnosis. The prevalence of osteoporosis is continuing to escalate with the increasing elderly population.

- Worldwide osteoporosis causes more than 8.9 million fractures annually, resulting in an osteoporotic fracture every 3 seconds.

- According to the recent statistics from International Osteoporotic Foundation (IOF), worldwide, 1 in 3 women and 1 in 5 men will experience osteoporotic fractures over the age of 50 years in their lifetime. Increased prevalence in women may be due to differences in peak bone mass and particularly to the loss of bone that occurs after menopause due to oestrogen deficiency.

- Fragility fractures are a leading cause of chronic disease morbidity. For instance in Europe, fragility fractures are the fourth leading cause after Ischaemic heart disease, Dementia and Lung cancer. However, they surpass chronic obstructive pulmonary disease and ischaemic stroke.

- According to the report by the US Surgeon General, approximately 10 million Americans over the age of 50 years have osteoporosis, with a further 34 million at risk of the disease. Osteoporotic fractures in the USA are extremely common, with an estimated 1.5 million suffering from fragility fractures each year. Of the estimated 10 million Americans with osteoporosis, about 8 million or 80% are women. Approximately, half of the women over the age of 50 years will break a bone because of osteoporosis.

(E) Prevalence, magnitude and burden of osteoporosis – Indian Scenario

- Primary data from India indicate a high prevalence rate of postmenopausal osteoporosis making it a major public health problem.

- In India, the prevalence of osteoporosis in postmenopausal women in various studies varies between 25% to 62%.

- Prevalence of low bone mass is more than 40% from the age of 40 and increases to

62% by age 60 and 80% by the age of 65 years. In 2013, study suggested that 50 million people in India had T-score less than -1.3.

- Recent data indicate that Indians have lower bone density than their North American and European counterparts. It is reported that osteoporotic fractures occur 10-20 years earlier in Indians compared to Caucasians. The probable reasons cited are genetic, environmental, early age at menopause and nutritional.

- Indian Council of Medical Research (ICMR) studies on three socio-economic groups at National Institute of Nutrition showed that after the age of 50 years, osteoporosis of the spine was only 16% in high income group (with calcium intake of 1000 mg) compared to low income group with 65% osteoporosis (calcium intake around 400).

- A review of the global Vitamin D status by International Osteoporotic Foundation (IOF) in 2009 underscores the fact that South Asia may be one of the worst affected regions in the world. Avoidances of sunlight exposure due to socio-economic reasons, environmental pollution, higher 25 (OH)-d-24-hydroxylase enzyme in Asian Indians are some of the reasons.

(F) Pathophysiology of osteoporosis:

Remodelling of bone

- The skeleton is composed of two types of bone
  - Cortical or compact bone.
  - Trabecular or calcaneus bone.

- Cortical or compact bone makes up to 80% of total body bone mass and predominates in skull and in shafts of long bones.
  Bone remodelling is a complex process directed towards renewal and repair of the skeleton.

- Since bone turnover is dependent on the surface area, it occurs more rapidly in trabecular bone than in cortical bone.

- Normal bone remodelling involves two types of cells:
  - Osteoblasts and
  - Osteoclasts

- Osteoclasts are primarily responsible for bone resorption. They resorb old bone and create a cavity on the bone surface.

- Osteoblasts, responsible for bone formation, fill the cavity with newly formed bone which then undergoes mineralization i.e. become impregnated with calcium. The complete cycle takes place in about 6 months.

Under normal conditions, the rate of bone resorption and formation is equal so that the total bone mass remains constant. The situation where bone formation cannot keep pace with bone resorption, osteoporosis results.

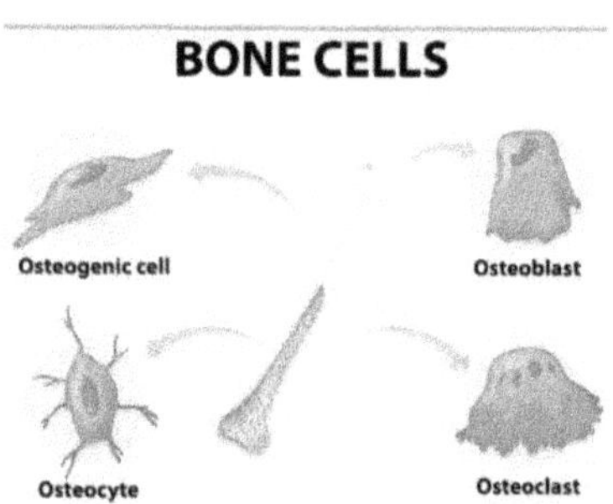

(G) Peak Bone Mass:

- All bones have a threshold value of bone mass below which fracture occurs.

- Peak bone mass is the result of interplay of various factors such as genetic, hormonal, racial, nutritional, lifestyle and physical exercise.
  Environmental factors modulate the expression of genetic potential to achieve peak bone mass.

- Actually lifestyle management with emphasis on nutrition and physical activity should start counselling from pre-pregnancy to postpartum period.
  Between the ages of 9-14 years, children will develop more bone than they will ever lose in their lifetime. They need help focusing on their bone health and more importantly on their bone development. Making the most of peak bone mass in younger age may help reduce the risk of osteoporosis and fractures in older age.

- By the age 18 years, children have developed 90% of their lifetime bone mass. By the age 30, most have reached peak bone mass, a maximum threshold that may protect them for several years but will require constant attention throughout mid and later stages of life.

- Adolescence is the critical period of skeletal development and peak bone mass. Evidence indicates that when peak bone mass increases by 5% during childhood and adolescence, the risk of osteoporotic fractures reduces by 40%; while when peak bone mass increases by 10%, this risk decreases by 50%. Therefore increased bone mass accumulation during this period is an effective way to maintain bone health in adulthood and prevent osteoporosis in older age groups.

- Sometimes after the age of 25 years, healthy men and women lose bone mass at the rate of 0.3 to 0.4% per year. After menopause, women lose bone mass at a far greater rate of 2-3% per year, after which the loss continues at a much slower rate.

- Men have much higher peak bone mass than women and therefore develop osteoporosis much later in life.

- Calcium supplementation seems to be the main nutritional determinant in bone mass acquisition. In children and adolescents in whom dietary calcium intake is deficient, calcium supplements as per RDA is recommended.

- Vitamin D has a major role in stimulating intestinal calcium absorption. In children and adolescents having an insufficient vitamin D status, vitamin D supplementation adequate enough for the age is recommended.

- Physical exercises, mainly weight-bearing activities, is a key factor for the acquisition and maintenance of bone mass. School authorities need to increase outdoor activities in children.

Determinants of Peak Bone Mass

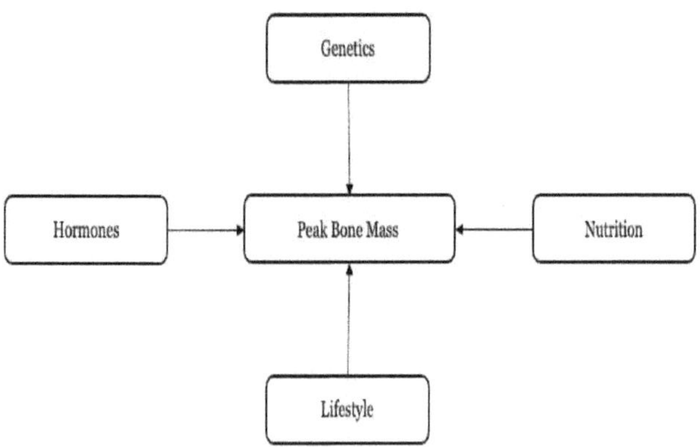

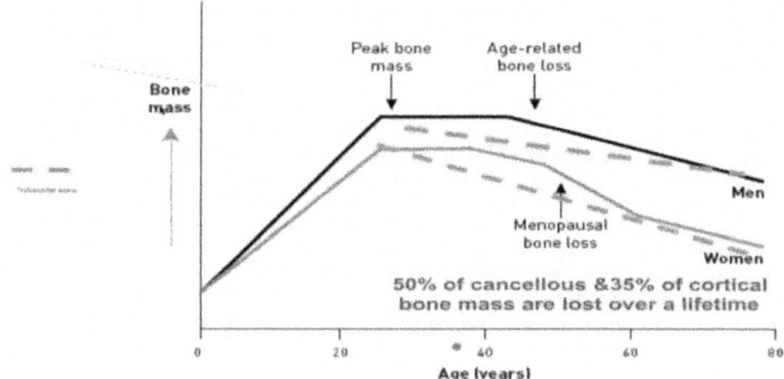

(H) Types of Osteoporosis:

Primary Osteoporosis

- Primary osteoporosis is used to define a condition in women or men in whom no pathogenic mechanism other than age-related sex steroid deficiency and aging can be correlated. Primary osteoporosis is of two types:

- **Primary osteoporosis type I or Postmenopausal osteoporosis:**
  Here the bone loss is the consequence of oestrogen deficiency. When oestrogen is lost from a woman's body after menopause, it triggers an inflammatory response. As a result, osteoclasts begin to work at an accelerated rate. This means one can start losing old bone faster than the osteoblast can replace it with new bone. Obvious result is bones get weaker, thinner and more vulnerable to trauma.

- **Primary osteoporosis type II or Senile osteoporosis:**
  Typically after the age of 70 years, kidneys become less able to convert Vitamin D into its active form. The reduced amount of Vitamin D in the body then hampers the absorption of dietary calcium. This causes your body to withdraw calcium from the bones leading to lower bone mass with consequent osteoporosis.

Secondary Osteoporosis

- Secondary osteoporosis is loss of bone or alterations in bone microarchitecture and leading to fragility fractures due to:
  - Underlying diseases
  - Medications
  - Lifestyle changes

- Although secondary osteoporosis is less common, it is becoming more frequently recognized, especially in postmenopausal women. In addition, although osteoporosis in postmenopausal women is usually linked to oestrogen deficiency, secondary causes are now being identified more often. In 20-30% of postmenopausal women and in more than 50% of males, osteoporosis is due to secondary causes.
- Secondary osteoporosis remains a diagnostic and therapeutic challenge. The underlying conditions are diverse and require specific diagnostic tests and treatment.

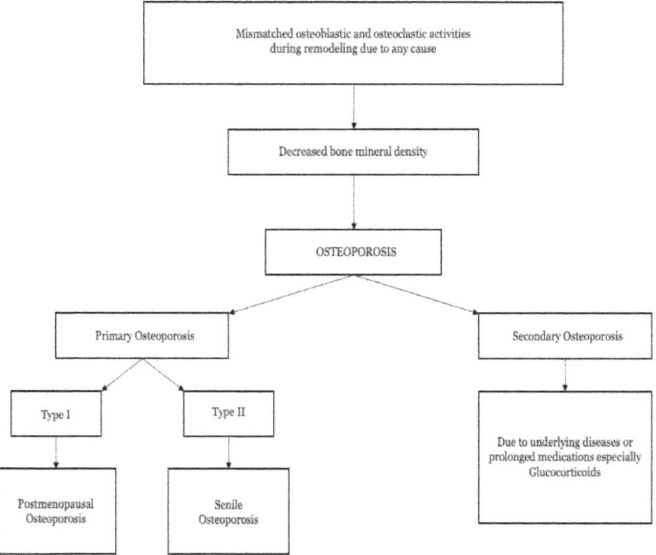

(I) Risk factors for osteoporosis:

There are many factors that can contribute to a greater likelihood of the development of osteoporosis. Some of these are non-modifiable risk factors while others are modifiable.

Non-modifiable Risk factors:

- **Age**
  Age is the single most important risk factor. Older persons suffer the most. Each decade beyond the fourth decade is 1.5 fold risk.

- **Gender**
  Women are much more likely to develop osteoporosis than men. This may be because of the low bone mass and oestrogen deficiency during menopause or similar such oestrogen deficiency conditions earlier.

- **Ethnicity**

Caucasians and Asian women are at higher risk.

- **Family History**

Osteoporosis and fracture risk may be due, in part, to heredity. People whose parents have the history of fractures also seem to have reduced bone mass and may be at risk.

- **Body frame size**

People with small body frames have a higher risk of osteoporosis.

Modifiable Risk Factors:

- **Nutritional factors**
    - Low calcium intake.
    - Vitamin D deficiency.
    - Eating disorders e.g. Anorexia Nervosa or Gastrointestinal surgeries.
    - Overall nutritional deficiency in the adolescent age group resulting in low bone mass.

- **Lifestyle**

  Lifestyle can influence risk of osteoporosis
    - Sedentary lifestyle.
    - Smoking.
    - Daily excessive consumption of alcohol.
    - Daily excessive consumption of caffeine.

- **Endocrine factors**
    - Estrogen deficiency due to any cause e.g. hypothalamic amenorrhea.
    - Thyroid disease – Risk is greater with untreated thyrotoxicosis.

- Overactive parathyroid and adrenal glands increase the risk of osteoporosis.

- **Medical conditions**
  - Celiac disease
  - Inflammatory bowel disease
  - Kidney or liver disease
  - Rheumatoid arthritis
  - Multiple myeloma
  - Cancer
  - Insulin dependent diabetes mellitus
  - HIV/AIDS

- **Drugs known to cause osteoporosis**
  - Glucocorticoids – Prednisolone
  - Progesterone – Depot Medroxyprogesterone Acetate (DMPA)
  - GnRH Agonist – Buserelin, Goserelin
  - Aromatase Inhibitors – Letrazol
  - Proton pump Inhibitors – Omeprazole or Pantaprazole
  - Lipase Inhibitors – Orlistat

(J) Screening, Diagnosis and Evaluation:

- Osteoporosis is asymptomatic unless fracture occurs. Early diagnosis in the asymptomatic period is important and timely management of osteoporosis will prevent the associated morbidity and mortality.

- Screening of osteoporosis of a large population group is not likely to be cost-effective in a country like India. So a more selective approach like targeted screening for disease detection is advocated.

- Risk assessment factors are derived by history, clinical examination and laboratory investigations. It is important to distinguish between those risk factors which lead to reduced bone mass from those which predisposes to osteoporotic fractures with BMD not in osteoporotic range.

Signs and Symptoms:

Osteoporosis is called "**Silent Disease**" because one may not notice any signs and symptoms unless the bone breaks. However, some signs and symptoms such as:

Receding gums

- Weaker hand grip strength
- More brittle fingernails
- Loss of height
- Stooped posture
- Back or neck pain
- Bone fracture with even lesser trauma

Physical Examination:

- Should include recording of height and weight annually. Also balance and gate to be checked.

- Get-up and Go test – by asking women to get-up from a chair without using their arms.

- Occiput to wall distance in standing position is ideally zero. Inability to touch occiput to the wall while standing indicates thoracic fracture.

- Inability to insinuate four fingers of the hand between the lower rib cage and anterior superior iliac crest indicates a lumbar fracture.

- Women presenting with fracture complain of severe pain, which is sudden in onset with minimal trauma.

- In Vitamin D deficiency, proximal muscle is affected more than the distal. So activities such as using a squatting toilet, climbing stairs and getting out of a lower heighted chair can be particularly difficult.

- Tenderness on the tibia and sternum can be elicited.

- Kyphosis and Dowager's hump are seen at late stages of osteoporosis.

Laboratory Studies:

- CBC, ESR
- Blood sugar – F, PP
- Serum Calcium
- Serum Albumin
- Serum Phosphorus preferably fasting
- Serum Creatinine
- Serum Alkaline Phosphatase
- Serum TSH
- 25 Hydroxy – Vitamin D
- X-Ray thoracolumbar region – lateral view
- PTH (based on clinical judgement)

Bone Mineral Density Test (BMD):

- Bone Mineral Density (BMD) test measures how much calcium and other types of minerals are in an area of your bone.

- Currently Dual Energy X-Ray Absorptiometry (DEXA) scan is **the gold standard** for clinical diagnosis of osteoporosis by bone densitometry.

- Bone densitometry is a widely accepted test for quantitative measurement of mineral density of the whole skeleton as well as specific sites, including those more prone to fractures.

- Diagnosis is based on central DEXA of spine, total hip and neck of femur. If this is not possible, lower $1/3^{rd}$ of radius (33%) is measured.

- The Caucasian female normative database is used as a reference for T-score.

- BMD measurements are quite specific (85%). The mortality adjusted lifetime risk of fracture for women with a T-score less than or equal to -2.5 is 65%.

- False positive high BMD may be due to fluorosis, which is prevalent in some parts of India.

- The number of available DEXA scanners are limited in India, with only 0.26 scanners for 1 million population.

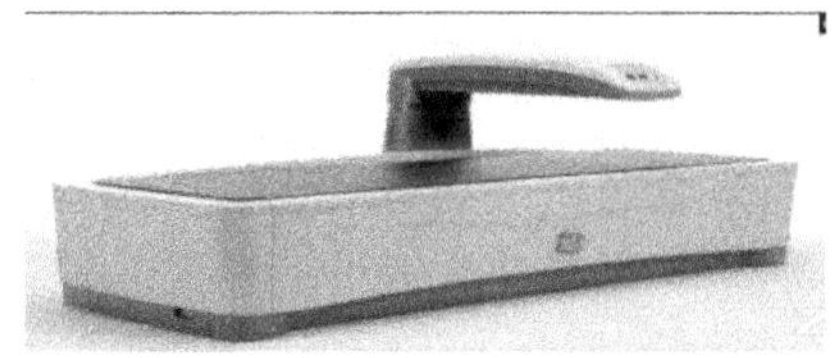

DEXA scanner

The results of the test are usually reported as:

1. **T-score** and
2. **Z-score**

T-score is a comparison of the patient's bone density with healthy young individuals of the same sex. T-score of -2.5 or less at the femoral neck defines osteoporosis. T-score is used to diagnose osteoporosis in postmenopausal women and men over the age of 50 years. (T-score is the number of units called standard deviations that a patient's bone density is above or below the average).

Z-score is a comparison with the bone density of the people of the same age and sex of the patient. Z-score of -2.5 or less should raise suspicion of a secondary cause of osteoporosis. Z-score is used to diagnose osteoporosis in children, teenagers, premenopausal women and younger men less than 50 years of age.

World Health Organization (WHO) criteria for diagnosis of osteoporosis:

- **Normal:** T-score above -1.0
- **Osteopenia or low bone mass:** T-score between -1 and -2.5
- **Osteoporosis:** T-score below -2.5
- **Severe osteoporosis:** T-score below -2.5 with fragility fracture

Interpretation of results:

- Osteopenia: > 2 fold increase in fracture, compared to normal
- Osteoporosis: > 4-5 fold increased risk of fracture
- Severe Osteoporosis: > 20 fold increased risk of fracture.

Indication for measurement of BMD:

American College of Obstetrics and Gynaecology (ACOG) recommends measurement of BMD in:

- All women aged 65 years and above.
- Women under 65 years with additional clinical risk factor.
- Alternatively, women under 65 years with FRAX 10 years risk of major osteoporotic fracture of 9.3% or higher.

  Measurement of BMD is also recommended before initiating pharmacotherapy for osteoporosis and to monitor the therapy.

  The National Osteoporotic Foundation (NOF) recommends repeat bone density every two years to assess the effect of therapy.

Contraindications of DEXA scan:

- Pregnancy is the absolute contraindication.
- Recently administered gastrointestinal contrast or radionuclides.
- Severe degenerative changes or fracture deformity in the measurement area.

- Implants, hardware devices or other foreign material in the measurement area.
- Calcium supplements or drugs that contain calcium should not be taken 24 hours before a densitometry test.

Other modalities:

Radiological Evaluation:

- Main radiographic features of generalised osteoporosis are increased radiolucency and cortical thinning.
- X-Ray abnormality is a feature of advanced bone disease.
- X-Ray of dorsal and lumbar spine is advised, both anteroposterior and lateral view. Vertebral fractures are mostly clinically silent, but their presence predisposes a person to further fragility fractures of vertebra or even hip.
- Radiologic technique cannot be used in monitoring drug therapy.
- Radiological evaluation is non-invasive, cheap but inconclusive in early osteoporosis.

Quantitative Ultrasound (QUS):

- QUS appears to be developing into an acceptable, low cost and readily accessible alternative to DEXA.
- Ultrasound can be used to measure the bone density of the heel. This may be useful to determine a person's fracture risk. However, it is used less frequently than DEXA because there are no guidelines for the use of

ultrasound measurements to diagnose osteoporosis or predict fracture risk.

- In places that do not have access to DEXA, ultrasound is an acceptable way to measure bone density.

Quantitative computerized tomography:

- This is a type of computed tomography (CT) that provides accurate measures of bone density in the spine. Although this may be an alternative to DEXA, it is seldomly used as it is expensive and requires a higher radiation dose.

MRI:

- Assesses 3-D picture of the bone.
- Differentiate between trabecular and cortical bone.
- Can diagnose micro fractures.
- Because of limited availability and high cost, it is not used.

(K) Risk Assessment Tools:

- Risk assessment tools can detect the risk of developing the disease in early stage in apparently healthy, asymptomatic individuals based upon the assessment of multiple variables.
- All of the available risk models have got advantages and disadvantages. Not a single model is appropriate for all patients.
- 48 tools identified, 20 validated but only 6 have been tested in population-based settings: 3 for risk assessment of osteoporosis and 3 for risk assessment of fracture.

Risk assessment tools for osteoporosis:

- OSTA (Osteoporosis Self-assessment Tool for Asians)
- ORAI (Osteoporosis Risk Assessment Instrument)
- SCORE (Simple Calculated Osteoporosis Risk Estimation)

Risk assessment tools for fracture:

- GARVAN
- FRAX
- QFracture

As each tool has its unique strengths and weaknesses, the aim is to monitor each individual scoring system's performance in order to develop tools, with better effective screening strategies, eventually improving the patient's care worldwide. Commonly used tools in practice are described here.

OSTA (Osteoporosis Self-assessment Tool for Asians):

- **The World Health Organization (WHO)** developed the OSTA score to identify women at risk of osteoporosis and is based simply on age and body weight.
- OSTA score can be calculated by subtracting age from weight and multiplying by 0.2.

OSTA = 0.2 (weight in kg – age in years)

Women are classified into three groups depending upon the risk: Low, Moderate and High.

Recommendation based on risks:

High risk patients

Measure BMD by DEXA and consider drug treatment.

(About 61% of individuals in the high risk group have osteoporosis)

Middle risk patients

Measure BMD by DEXA and consider drug treatment if BMD is low.

(About 15% of individuals in the moderate risk group have osteoporosis)

Low risk patients

It is not necessary to measure BMD unless other risk factors are present.

(Only about 3% of individuals in the low risk group have osteoporosis)

Efficacy:

- Test sensitivity: 91.1%
- Test specificity: 45%

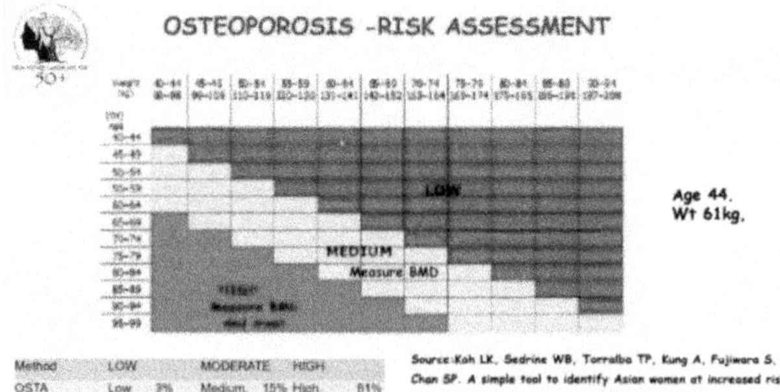

SCORE (Simple Calculated Osteoporosis Risk Estimation)

This scoring system includes age, race, weight, estrogen use, history of arthritis and history of non-traumatic fractures.

How to calculate the score?

- o Race no black: 5 points
- o Rheumatoid Arthritis: 4 points
- o Fractures after the age 45 of wrist, hip or rib: 4 points per fracture
- o Age over 65: Calculate 3 x (1st digit of age) For example for age 70: 3 x 7 = 21

Weight: Calculate (-1 x weight in pounds) / 10
For example for weight 200 pounds: -20.

- o Estrogen therapy never used: 1

Interpretation:

- **Low risk**: Score of 6 and below.
- **Moderate risk**: Score between 7 and 15.
- **Severe risk**: Score of 16 and above.

Recommendation:

- o BMD with DXA is recommended if score of 6 and above and if the BMD is low, drug therapy may be considered accordingly.

Efficacy:

- Test sensitivity: 91%
- Test specificity: 40%

FRAX: WHO Fracture Risk Assessment Tool

- Online-Tool : (http://www.shef.ac.uk/FRAX)

- WHO collaborating centre at Sheffield UK released FRAX in 2008 – a computer-based algorithm that calculates individualized 10 year probability of hip and major osteoporotic fractures.
- Currently 71 models are available worldwide in 66 countries covering more than 80% of world population.
- It is available in 35 languages.
- 3 million visits annually on this website.
- FRAX for the Indian population is also available now.
- In view of the limited availability of DEXA machines in India, it will be helpful to use FRAX without BMD in the Indian context.
- Heterogeneity in different regions of the country and the prevalence of nutritional and other risk factors unique to the Indian population has not been considered in the calculation of FRAX.
- FRAX is country-specific, and until more Indian data is available on the prevalence of osteoporotic fractures and mortality rates, the usage of FRAX in the Indian context for uniform guidance on intervention threshold is to be applied cautiously.

Strength of FRAX:

- ✓ FRAX may have great potential to assist the clinical decision making and ultimately in improving patient outcome.
- ✓ It is a tool validated on 250,000 patient years of follow-up.
- ✓ It is an additional tool for fracture prediction with and without BMD.

- ✓ Aids in decision making in cases of osteopenia.
- ✓ Simple screening test using BMI instead of BMD thus avoiding unnecessary investigations.
- ✓ The FRAX platform is global and subject to modifications.

Limitations of FRAX:

- ✓ Risk factors are dichotomous, involving a Yes/No response, can result in either over or underestimation of fracture risk.
- ✓ FRAX does not take into account dose-response relationships. For example, FRAX does not make a difference between single versus multiple fractures.
- ✓ The increased subsequent fracture risk after initial fracture is considered constant over time in FRAX.
- ✓ Poor definition of secondary osteoporosis.
- ✓ Internet access required.
- ✓ There may be racial or ethnic differences that influence fracture risk not taken into account by FRAX.

Valuable tool if used appropriately.

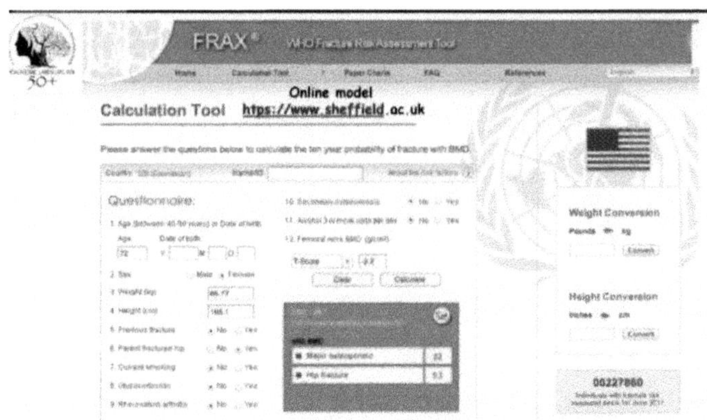

(L) Bone Turnover Markers (BTMs):

- ✓ Bone turnover markers are blood and urine tests that detect a series of protein or protein derivatives released during bone remodelling by osteoblasts and osteoclasts.
- ✓ Bone turnover markers are not a part of routine tests to be used for clinical diagnosis of osteoporosis.
- ✓ Several tests can act as bone turnover markers. They are classified as:

Markers of bone formation.
Markers of bone resorption.

A summary list of bone formation markers is as follows:

- o Serum total alkaline phosphatase.
- o Serum bone-specific alkaline phosphatase.
- o Serum osteocalcin.
- o Serum type 1 procollagen (C-Terminal / N-terminal) : C1NP or P1NP

A summary list of bone resorption markers is as follows:

- Urinary total pyridinoline (PYD)
- Urinary free deoxypyridinoline (DPD)
- Urinary collagen type 1 cross-linked N-telopeptide (NTX)
- Urinary or serum collagen type 1 cross-linked C-telopeptide (CTX)
- Bone sialoprotein (BSP)
- Tartrate-resistant acid phosphatase 5b

To be more specific, use markers for bone resorption when a patient is on antiresorptive therapy while bone formation markers when on anabolic agents.

Timing of sample:

Serum – Morning (before 9 am) after an overnight fast.
Urine – Either first or second morning void, with creatinine correction after an overnight fast.
(Try to use the same laboratory services and the same essay or method of monitoring.)

Intervals of measurement:

Resorption markers: Before starting treatment and 3-6 months after the treatment has been initiated.

Formation markers: Before starting treatment and 6 months after the treatment has been initiated.

Interpretation of results:

- The results in markers during treatment should be interpreted in terms of the 'Least Significant Change' (LSC). LSC is the minimum change that must be seen in the results to be at least 95% sure that change is real and not caused by pre-analytical and analytical factors.

- LSC is about 25% for most bone formation markers and 40-65% for most resorption factors.

- When there is little or no change in markers during treatment, then check for:
  - ✓ Whether patient is taking prescribed medicines or not and
  - ✓ Rule out secondary causes of osteoporosis.

Diagnosis of osteoporosis is not based on evaluation of bone markers. BMD assessment is still the standard criteria for diagnosis and evaluation. The combined use of BMD measurement and bone markers is likely to improve the assessment of risk of fractures.

(M) Management of Osteoporosis:

Osteoporosis and broken bones are not part of normal aging. There are many things one can do to protect bone health throughout one's life. It is never too early or late to improve bone health.

From intrauterine life, infant life, childhood, early adolescence, late adolescence – all stages of life are important to increase peak bone mass.

Once optimum 'peak bone mass' is achieved up to 25-30 years of age; chances of osteoporosis and osteoporosis related fractures especially in old age will also be reduced unless there are other risk factors.

A population-based and a personalized approach is to be implemented to prevent and treat postmenopausal osteoporosis. It is better to understand the term prevention and treatment in the context of osteoporosis.

Prevention of Osteoporosis:

The term prevention is used here to denote prevention of further bone loss in postmenopausal women with established osteopenia (T-score between -1 and -2.5) thus preventing progress to osteoporosis. Prevention strategies include:

- **Substrates for bone nutrition:**
  - ✓ Healthy and balanced diet with plenty of fresh fruits, green vegetables and whole grains.
  - ✓ Calcium.
  - ✓ Vitamin D.
  - ✓ Vitamin K.
  - ✓ Proteins.

- **Exercise:**
  - ✓ Weight-bearing exercises.
  - ✓ Strength training.
  - ✓ Flexibility exercises.
  - ✓ Stability and balance exercises.

- **Lifestyle modifications:**
  - ✓ Stop smoking.

- ✓ Limit alcohol.
- ✓ Limit caffeine.
- ✓ Limit salt.
- ✓ Limit red meat.

Calcium:

Calcium is a mineral most often associated with healthy bones and teeth. It also plays an important role in blood clotting, helping muscles to contract, regulating normal heart rhythm and nerve functions. About 99% of the body's calcium is stored in bones and teeth, while the remaining 1% is found in blood, muscles and other tissues.

Best way to get optimum calcium daily:

- The best way to get optimum calcium every day is to eat a variety of healthy food from all different kinds of food groups. Getting optimum Vitamin D every day from natural sunlight is important to help the body absorb and use calcium from food.
- Dairy products have the highest calcium content. Dairy products include milk, yogurt and cheese. A large cup of milk contains 300 mg of calcium. The calcium content is same for skimmed milk, low fat and whole milk.
- Dark green leafy vegetables contain high amount of calcium. Broccoli, Kale and Collards are all good sources of calcium, especially when eaten raw or lightly steamed. (Boiling vegetables may take out much of their mineral content).
- A serving of canned Salmon or Sardines have about 200 mg of calcium. Calcium is found in soft bones of the fish.

- Cereals, pasta, bread and fruit juices fortified with calcium add calcium to the diet.

Recommended Dietary Allowance (RDA) of calcium for Indian woman:

Group	Calcium (mg)
Adult woman	600 – 1000
Pregnancy	1200
Lactation	1200
Postmenopausal woman	800 – 1200

Source: National Institute of Nutrition/Indian

Council of Medical Research NIN/ICMR 2020):

Is it necessary to take calcium supplements?

Calcium is best absorbed through the food we eat and the beverages we drink. For most healthy patients, it is important to eat a well-balanced diet instead of relying on supplements. But even if you eat healthy balanced diet, you may find it difficult to get recommended daily calcium in following situations, if you:

- ✓ Follow a vegan diet and avoid dairy products or
- ✓ Have a lactose intolerance and avoid dairy products or
- ✓ Consume large amount of proteins or sodium which can cause your body to excrete more calcium or
- ✓ Have certain bowel or digestive diseases that decreases your ability to absorb

calcium such as inflammatory bowel disease or celiac disease or

- ✓ Receiving long term treatment with corticosteroids.

(In these situations, calcium supplements may help you meet your daily calcium requirements.)

Which calcium supplements/compounds to be preferred?

- Several different kinds of calcium compounds are used in calcium supplements. Each compound contains varying amounts of calcium – referred to as '**Elemental Calcium**'. It is this 'Elemental Calcium' which is important because it is the actual amount of calcium your body absorbs for bone health and other health benefits. Again the cost factor needs to be taken into consideration.

Calcium supplements available in market are:

Calcium compounds	% of elemental calcium	mg elemental calcium/1gm
Calcium Carbonate	40%	400
Calcium Citrate	21%	210
Calcium Citrate Maleate	26%	260
Calcium Acetate	25%	250
Calcium Lactate	13%	130
Calcium Gluconate	9%	90
Calcium Orotate	10%	100

- Two main forms of calcium compounds are calcium carbonate and calcium citrate. **Calcium carbonate is the cheapest and contains 40% elemental calcium and therefore a first good choice**. Calcium carbonate dissolves better in an acidic environment, so it should be taken with meals. Following situations are unfavourable for acidic environment resulting in defective absorption of calcium carbonate:
    - ✓ Women who are on antacids to reduce acid to get relief from acidity, heartburn.
    - ✓ Those who have had intestinal bypass surgery.
    - ✓ 65 years and above.

(In such situations where calcium carbonate absorption is reduced, calcium citrate compounds are preferable. Calcium citrate can be taken at any time because they do not require an acidic environment to dissolve. The disadvantage with citrate compound is that it is little costly and more tablets need to be taken as elemental calcium is only 21%).

How much is a single dose of calcium at a time?

- Higher the one time calcium dose, lesser is the absorption. For maximum absorption, no more than 500 mg of calcium should be taken in a single dose. If your requirement is more than 500 mg daily, then it should be taken in divided doses, at least 4 hours apart.

Overdoses of calcium:

- Dietary calcium is generally safe, but more is not necessarily better and excessive intake of calcium does not produce extra bone protection.

- Adults aging between 19 and 50 should not take more than 2500 mg calcium daily (total calcium including dietary and supplementary).

- Adults over 50 years should not exceed 2000 mg total calcium per day.

- Too much calcium daily in the form of supplements might have some health risks.

Risk associated with excessive calcium:

- Increased heart attack risk as calcium tends to build up in coronaries. (more research is required to establish a link)
- Increased prostate cancer risk (more research is required to establish a link).
- Increased risk of kidney stones.

Interactions of calcium with other medications:

Calcium can reduce the absorption of following medications if taken at same time with:

- Bisphosphonates
- Thyroid medications
- Certain seizure medications e.g. phenytoin
- Calcium channel blocker
- Iron, zinc, magnesium

Dietary calcium restriction is no longer recommended for patients with hypercalciuria. But the data on supplemental calcium intake is currently controversial. In cases where calcium supplementation is medically necessary, patients should be encouraged to take their calcium supplements with meal and should be monitored by hypercalciuria. It is also important to drink plenty of water to dilute substances in urine.

Vitamin-D:

Role of Vitamin-D:

- Estrogen increases activity of 1,25-hydroxylase which ultimately activates vitamin D. Deficiency of oestrogen in menopause can trigger symptoms of vitamin D deficiency.

- It prevents serotonin depletion thus reducing the severity of hot flashes.
- It helps us to keep muscles strong and to reduce the risk of falling.

- It reduces the risk of cardiovascular and metabolic diseases.

- It positively affects cognition and mood.

- Vitamin D also regulates many other cellular functions in the body. Its anti-inflammatory, antioxidant and neuroprotective properties support immune health, muscle health and brain cell activity.

- Vitamin D deficiency is associated with increased susceptibility to respiratory tract infections.

Do Indians have sufficient levels of Vitamin D?

Retrospective analysis of records of 4624 patients across India have shown that:

- Up to 76.9% of Indians have insufficient vitamin D levels.
- Highest level of vitamin D deficiency in the age group 18-30 years.
- Vitamin D deficiency is marginally higher in males (77.3 %) than females (76.5 %).

Probable reasons for Vitamin D deficiency in Indians?

- Diet – very few foods are rich in vitamin D. Dietary sources of vitamin D are predominantly non-vegetarian (salmon, egg yolks). Only vegetarian sources are sun-exposed mushrooms and fortified foods.

- Increased melanin content of skin of Indians.

- Inadequate sunlight exposure.

- Lack of vitamin D fortified food available in India as against in western countries.

Vitamin D levels for diagnosis:

(Institute of Medicine Committee/Endocrine Society of clinical guidelines):

- **<20 ng/ml - Deficiency**
- **21-29 ng/ml - Insufficiency**

- **>30 ng/ml - Sufficient (normal)**

Optimum level of serum 25 (OH) D is 30-60 ng/ml as per US Endocrine Society. To maintain serum 25 (OH) D level in optimum range and also in the background of widespread vitamin D deficiency, it is prudent to adopt the US Endocrine Society RDA for Vitamin D 2011.

US Endocrine Society RDA 2011 for Vitamin D

Life stage group	RDA (IU)	Upper limit
Adults 18 yrs and above	1500 - 2000	10000
Pregnancy and lactation	*1500 - 2000*	10000

Many other countries around the world and some professional societies have somewhat different guidelines for vitamin D intakes. These differences are as result of an incomplete understanding of the biology and clinical implications of vitamin D. The dose should not exceed 4000 IU/day and hypercalciuria have been reported when the dose exceeds 10000 IU/day.

Sources of Vitamin D:

Ultraviolet rays of sunlight.

- Vitamin D is made in the skin when the skin is exposed to ultraviolet rays of sunlight. Only a limited number of foods contain vitamin D, so exposing skin to sunlight is how we get 70-80% of vitamin D our body needs.

- The type of vitamin D made in the skin is called vitamin D3 (Cholecalciferol) and the form of vitamin D that you get through your diet which is closely related to a molecule of plant origin known as vitamin D2 (Ergocalciferol).
- **How much sun exposure is needed?**

    - To get vitamin D, generally, one should expose 15-30% of the body surface area (face, neck, both arms and forearms) without sunscreen for at least 20-30 minutes outside in peak sun hours between 10 am to 2 pm daily and taking care not to have sunburns.

    - Unfortunately, sunlight is not always a reliable source of Vitamin D. Vitamin D formation depends upon skin type, geographical location and the season. Fair-skinned individuals and those who are younger convert sunlight into Vitamin D better than those who are darker skinned and over 50 years of age. Because many of us spend most of our time indoors, low levels of vitamin D have become a worldwide problem and there is concern that this is having a negative impact on bone health.

Sources of Vitamin D in food

Very few foods are naturally rich in vitamin D. Therefore in some countries, certain foods and drinks such as margarine, breakfast cereals and orange juice are fortified with vitamin D. Natural food sources of vitamin D includes:

- Oily fish (salmon, herring, mackerel)
- Liver
- Eggs

Need for Vitamin D supplements:

Intake of Vitamin D from natural sources has practical limitations. Hence it is recommended to use Vitamin D as supplements so as to maintain serum 25 (OH) D level at optimum level (between 30-60 ng/ml).

Oral preparations (Cholecalciferol):

- Oral tablets – 1000 IU and 2000 IU

- Oral tablets/powder, granules in sachet – 60,000 IU

Injectable preparations:

- In the doses of 300000 and 600000 IU/ampule

Management of Vitamin D deficiency:

- Oral Cholecalciferol (Vitamin D3) in the form of tablets/powder/granules 60,000 IU once a week for 8 weeks preferably with milk. OR

- Injection of 600000 IU intramuscular (Not to be repeated before 3 months and may be given after confirmation of persisting low levels of Vitamin D).

Maintenance therapy:

- Oral tablets 1500 – 2000 IU/day. OR
- Oral tablets/powder/granules 60,000 IU once a month in summer and twice a month in winter. OR
- Injection of Cholecalciferol 300000 IU Intramuscular twice a year or Injection Cholecalciferol 600000 IU once a year.

Calcitriol:

Calcitriol is actually the most active form of Vitamin D (100 times more active than 25 (OH) D3). It has a very short half-life period of about a few hours. Calcitriol is used to treat low levels of calcium and bone disease in patients whose kidneys and parathyroid glands are not working normally. It is also used to treat secondary hyperparathyroidism. Calcitriol works by helping the body to use more of calcium found in foods and supplements and regulating the body's production of parathyroid hormone.

Vitamin K:

- Research has suggested that vitamin K plays a key role in controlling bone metabolism because it is essential for synthesizing osteocalcin, an important protein for maintaining bone health.

- Vitamin K comes in two forms:

Vitamin K1 (Phyllo Quinone)
Vitamin K2 (Mena Quinone)

- Vitamin K1 is found in green, leafy and cruciferous vegetables such spinach, kale, broccoli and Brussel's sprouts.

- Vitamin K2 is primarily produced by bacteria in the gut but is also found in small quantities in grass fed meats and dairy products. Greater quantities are found in fermented foods like natto – A Japanese soybean product.

- Studies so far have shown mixed results for supplements of vitamin K1 and K2. Some have found improved bone mineral density, a few showed decreased risk fracture and others found no additional benefit to bone health.

- The US Food and Drug Administration so far has not authorized health claims on labels for products containing Vitamin K2. Until there is more evidence to support taking supplements, focus should be on getting a balanced diet in order to get the Vitamin K1 and K2 that our bones need.

- Recommended dose of Vitamin K is 120-150 mcg daily. Avoid taking too much vitamin K as high doses can cause flushing and sweating.

Proteins and other nutrients:

- In addition to calcium in the presence of adequate vitamin D, dietary protein is a key nutrient for bone health across the lifespan and therefore has a function in prevention of osteoporosis. Protein makes up roughly 50% of the volume of the bone.

- It is important for the adolescent age group to eat enough protein-rich foods so that their bones develop and grow optimally. In seniors, protein plays a role in preserving bone and muscle mass.

- Animal sources of proteins include red meat, fish, eggs and dairy foods whereas vegetable sources of proteins include legumes (e.g. lentils, kidney beans), soya products (e.g. tofu), grains, nuts and seeds.

- The current recommended daily allowance for healthy adults is 1 gm protein per kg body weight. Protein intake stimulates the release of Insulin-like growth factor-1 (IGF-1) which increases muscle mass and bone growth.

- Low protein intake (<0.8 grams/kg body weight/day) is often observed in patients with hip fractures. Lower protein intake leads to lower IGF-1 which in turn leads to a lower bone mass. This could result in higher fracture risk.

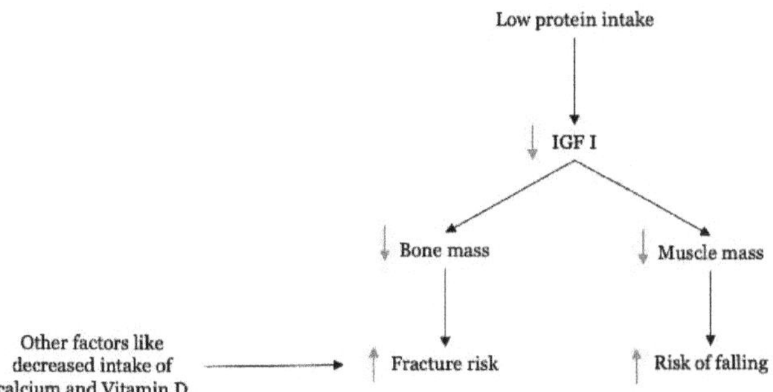

Exercise:

- Osteoporosis is the major cause of disability in older women. Osteoporosis often results in fractures in the hip and spine which can severely impair mobility and independence.

- Certain types of exercises strengthen bones and muscles while others are designed to improve balance which can help prevent falls.

- There is **no 'one-size-fits-all'** prescription as far as recommending exercise for a woman with osteoporosis is concerned. Exercise with osteoporosis means finding the safest and enjoyable activities for the overall benefits. Hence, it is always better to visit healthcare providers who may do BMD measurement and fitness assessment for prescribing right exercises.

- It is never too late to start exercising.

- Following types of exercises are usually recommended:
    - ✓ Weight-bearing aerobic exercises
    - ✓ Strength training exercises
    - ✓ Flexibility exercises
    - ✓ Stability and balance exercises

- Weight-bearing exercises like walking, jogging, dancing, stair climbing, gardening, low impact aerobics can work directly on the bones of legs, hips and lower spine to slow mineral loss. They also provide cardiovascular benefits.

- Swimming and cycling are excellent for other health benefits, but they do not promote bone health.

- Strength training includes the use of free weights or the use of resistant bands. It strengthens all major muscle groups, especially spinal muscles important for posture and also helps to maintain bone density.

- Flexibility exercises include moving joints through their full range of motion. It helps in preventing restricted movements.

- Stability and balance exercises help muscles to work together in a way that keeps the body more stable and less likely to fall. Simple exercises such as standing on one leg or movement based exercises such a 'Tai chi' can improve stability and balance.

High-impact exercises, bending and twisting exercises can lead to fractures in weakened bones. Hence choose exercises with slow, controlled movements.

Lifestyle modifications:

Stop smoking:

Smoking affects the body's ability to absorb calcium leading to lower bone density and weaker bones. Nicotine slows the production of the osteoblasts that are so crucial for bone healing. Smoking appears to break down oestrogen – a key ingredient in building and maintaining a healthy skeleton.

Limit alcohol:

Drink alcohol in moderation, if somebody is having a habit of drinking. Excessive alcohol increases the risk of osteoporosis. Drink not more than 1-2 standard drinks per day and have at least two alcohol-free days in a week.

Limit Caffeine:

According to **the National Osteoporotic Federation (NOF)** drinking more than 2-3 cups of caffeinated coffee or tea may decrease calcium absorption and contribute to bone loss. A cup (150 ml) of brewed coffee contains 80-120 mg caffeine and instant coffee 50-65 mg, while tea contains 30-65 mg. Generally low doses (20-150 mg) of caffeine produce mild positive effects like a feeling of well-being, alertness and energy. High dose (>200mg) can produce negative effects like nervousness and anxiety.

Limit Salt:
Sodium increases the excretion of calcium from the body. Their salt consumption should be limited to 1 teaspoonful (4-5 gms) per day.

Limit liver and fish liver oil intake:
Vitamin A is essential for healthy bones, skin, teeth and eyes. But too much of vitamin A may negatively affect bone health. **The United Kingdom's National Health Services** advise not to eat liver for more than a week in a month. (Liver is a rich source of vitamin A and some people regularly eat liver). One should also avoid excessive fish liver oil and nutritional supplements containing retinol.

Limit red meat:
In western countries animal meat remains the main common source of dietary proteins. Meat protein contains a high amount of sulphur containing amino acids. To tackle this influx, the body dissolves calcium from the bones and releases it into the bloodstream, which is hazardous for patients with osteoporosis.

Treatment of Osteoporosis:

- Treatment is defined as a reduction in fracture risk in postmenopausal women with already established osteoporosis.
- Apart from pharmacotherapy, it includes all the things covered in the preventive

part and also fracture prevention strategies due to fall.

Pharmacotherapy:

- Antiresorptive agents (Drugs which inhibit bone resorption)
- Bone anabolic agents (Drugs which stimulate bone formation)

Indications for pharmacotherapy:

AACE/ACE recommends that pharmacological treatment should be initiated for:

- Patients with osteopenia or low bone mass and a history of fragility fractures at the hip or spine.

- Patients with a T-score of -2.5 or less in the lumbar spine, femoral neck, total hip or 33% radius despite the absence of fracture.

- Patients with a T-score between -1.0 and -2.5, if the FRAX 10 year probability for a major osteoporotic fracture is greater than 20% or for a hip fracture is greater than 3%.

Antiresorptive therapy:

- Bisphosphonates
- SERMS
- MHT
- Denosumab
- Tibolone
- TSEC
- Calcitonin

Bisphosphonates:

- Bisphosphonates are recommended as first line drugs for treating osteoporosis.

- Bisphosphonates bind with high affinity to the mineral matrix of the bone and inhibit osteoclast resorption of the bone, with proven efficiency in the prevention of vertebral and nonvertebral fractures.

- Bisphosphonates can safely be given in women with risk of breast cancer.

- Oral bisphosphonates should be administered with a full glass of water in the morning on an empty stomach 30 minutes prior to a meal or other medications. (60 minutes in case of Ibandronate). Patients should remain in an upright position either sitting or standing for at least 30 minutes post-dose to prevent oesophageal irritation. Because the most common adverse effect of oral therapy is **oesophageal and gastric irritation** and is contraindicated in women with oesophageal abnormalities.

- In recommended doses bisphosphonate related **osteonecrosis of the jaw (ONJ)** is a rare complication. Routine dental check-up and treatment with vitamin D and calcium deficiency should be corrected before starting therapy.

- There is a possible risk of '**atypical femoral fracture**' which limits its use for 5 years. It is recommended to consider a '**drug free holiday**' after 3-5 years of therapy. Therapy can be stopped after 3-5 years in patients with low risk of fracture with a BMD approaching normal. Duration of treatment and length of drug holiday should be individualized based on the risk and benefits.

- In patients with high fracture risk, suggested duration of treatment is 10 years. Stay off bisphosphonates for 1-2 years, alternative medications e.g. Raloxifene or Teriparatide may be given during the holidays.

Doses and routes of administration of different bisphosphonates:

Tab Alendronate

- 5-10 mg/day, 70 mg/week, 150 mg/month
- Prevention of vertebral fractures 50%, hip fracture 51-56%, nonvertebral 49%.

Tab Risedronate

- 5 mg/day, 35 mg/week, 150 mg/month
- Prevention of vertebral fractures 41-49%, hip fracture 30%, nonvertebral 36%.

Injection Zoledronate

- 5mg I.V. over at least 15 minutes once yearly.
- Prevention of vertebral fractures 70%, hip 41%, and nonvertebral 25%.
- Anaphylaxis: even fatal events can occur.

Tab/Inj. Ibandronate

- 150 mg/day orally, 3 mg I.V. / every 3 months.

Selective Estrogen Receptor Modulators

(SERMs):

- SERMs are agents which interact with oestrogen receptors but have different oestrogenic actions in different tissues. They are oestrogen-agonist at bone while oestrogen-antagonist at breast.

- SERMs may be considered potential therapeutic agents for the prevention of postmenopausal osteoporosis.

Raloxifene:

- Raloxifene may be considered as a first line drug along with bisphosphonates.

- Raloxifene 60 mg/day improves and preserves bone density at spine (2.6%) and hip (2.1%) after 4 years with a simultaneous reduction by 76% in the risk of invasive breast cancer.

- Raloxifene has been shown to be beneficial in reducing vertebral fracture risk by 60% in postmenopausal women with osteoporosis and 47% in postmenopausal women with osteopenia over 3 years. Antifracture property on risk is lacking.

- **Raloxifene can be used as therapy for the prevention and treatment of osteoporosis especially for women with an increased risk of breast cancer.**

- **The risk of menopausal hot flashes and deep vein thrombosis (DVT)** are potential factors to be considered before choosing Raloxifene.

Bazedoxifene:

- Bazedoxifene is a third generation SERM that has been purposefully synthesized to improve skeletal and lipid parameters.

- Bazedoxifene acts as oestrogen-receptor on bones while oestrogen-receptor antagonists on breast tissue and uterus.

- Indicated for the following conditions alone or in combination with conjugated oestrogens in women with uterus.
    - ✓ Treatment of moderate to severe vasomotor symptoms associated with menopause.
    - ✓ Prevention of postmenopausal osteoporosis:

(Dose is 20-40 mg orally/day.)

Menopausal Hormone Therapy (MHT):

MHT is used for the prevention of fractures in postmenopausal women with osteoporosis, but after fulfilling following criteria **(Endocrine Society 2019)**

- ✓ Women under 60 years of age and <10 years postmenopausal.
- ✓ With bothersome vasomotor symptoms.
- ✓ Those in whom Bisphosphonates and Denosumab are not appropriate.
- ✓ No other contraindications to MHT.

Prevents vertebral fractures 30-70%, hip 40%, nonvertebral 27%.

Denosumab:

- Denosumab is a fully human monoclonal anti-receptor activator of nuclear factor Kappa-B ligand antibody, which inhibits the activity of osteoclast resulting in an antiresorptive effect with a significant increase in bone mineral density.

- It increases both trabecular and cortical bone strength. Prevents vertebral fractures 68%, hip 40%, nonvertebral 20%.

- **It can be used in patients with eGFR < 30 ml/min where bisphosphonates are contraindicated.**

- Discontinuation can result in rebound bone resorption.
  (Dose – Inj. Denosumab 60 mg subcutaneously once in 6 months.)

Tibolone:

- Tibolone is a **Selective Tissue Estrogenic Activity Regulator (STEAR)**. Post absorption, its metabolites have estrogenic, progestogenic and androgenic properties. The estrogenic effects are seen mainly in bone, brain and vaginal tissues and are responsible for control of vasomotor symptoms, prevention of bone loss and to improve libido.

- Tibolone increases lumbar spine and total hip BMD to a significantly greater extent than Raloxifene.

- **Tibolone may be preferable to MHT in symptomatic menopausal women with mammographically dense breast shadow.**

- It prevents vertebral fractures in 50%, hip in 26% and nonvertebral fractures in 26%.

- **Tibolone should not be used in breast cancer survivors as it increases the recurrence risk.**

- It is contraindicated in patients who have strong risks for stroke and over 60 years of age.

- It is approved in 90 countries to treat menopausal symptoms and in 45 countries to prevent osteoporosis.

- Single oral daily dose of 2.5 mg, even 1.25 mg has been found equally effective.

- When tibolone is used as an add back therapy with GnRH analog for treatment of endometriosis and fibroids, for control of vasomotor symptoms, there is added advantage of an increase in BMD.

Tissue Selective Estrogen Complex (TSEC):

- TSEC concept: The combination of a SERM with other oestrogens to achieve optimal clinical results based on their tissue selective activity profile.
- The first TSEC in clinical development partners, bazedoxifene (BZA), a SERM with a unique endometrial and breast safety profile, is used with conjugated oestrogens (CEE).
- BZA 20 mg/CEE 0.45 mg and BZA 20 mg/CEE 0.625 mg have shown efficacy in reducing the severity of hot flashes and maintaining bone mass while protecting the endometrium and the breast.

Calcitonin:

- Calcitonin is a hormone that helps regulate how the body uses calcium. It is produced by special cells in the thyroid gland called C-cells.

- Calcitonin binds to calcitonin receptors on osteoclasts to inhibit bone resorption.

- Reduces the risk of vertebral fractures, no proven benefit for hip or nonvertebral fractures.

- Dose: 200 IU intranasal spray daily or 100 IU subcutaneous inj.

- Other effects include possible analgesic effects.

Bone Anabolic Therapy:

Teriparatide:

- Teriparatide is a synthetic form of natural human hormone called parathyroid hormone (PTH)

- It is the only agent that increases new bone formation (Anabolic). It works by causing the body to build new bone and by increasing bone strength and density.

- FDA approved it in 2002 for severe osteoporosis.

Indications:

✓ Treatment of osteoporosis in postmenopausal women with high risk of fracture, including those with very low BMD (T-score worse than -3.0).
✓ With previous vertebral fracture or other osteoporotic features.
✓ Those patients intolerant of or unresponsive to antiresorptive therapy.
✓ Glucocorticoid-induced osteoporosis.

Administration:

✓ Teriparatide administration is via subcutaneous injection into the abdominal wall or anterior thigh.
✓ The dosage is 20 mcg per day.
✓ **Maximum duration of therapy is limited to 2 years because of theoretical risk of osteosarcoma.**

- ✓ May be followed by antiresorptive therapy if required.
- ✓ No advantage of combined anabolic and anti-receptive therapy.

Contraindications:

- ✓ Hypersensitivity to Teriparatide.
- ✓ Increased basal risk for osteosarcoma like Paget disease of bone, history of primary or secondary skeletal malignancy, history of ionizing radiation involving the skeleton.
- ✓ Hypercalcemia.
- ✓ Hypercalciuria and or urolithiasis which promotes urinary stones.
- ✓ Have severe kidney or liver problems.
- ✓ Pregnancy or breastfeeding.

(Patients taking Teriparatide are also prescribed with calcium and vitamin D supplements.)

Side-effects:

- ✓ Leg cramp
- ✓ dizziness.

(N) Glucocorticoid induced Osteoporosis:

- ✓ Glucocorticoid induced osteoporosis is the common cause of secondary osteoporosis and is an iatrogenic disease.

- ✓ Fracture risk is correlated with the dose and duration of glucocorticoid administration. 7.5 mg or more prednisolone daily for an anticipated duration of 3 or more months and even daily doses as low as 2.5 mg for 6 or more months has been shown to increase the risk of bone loss and subsequent risk of fracture.

- ✓ Inhaled glucocorticoid below 400 mcg/day and usage of budesonide or fluticasone seemed to have minimal systemic effects compared to betnesol.

- ✓ Bone loss occurs most rapidly in the first 6 months after starting oral steroids. After 12 months of chronic steroid use, there is slower loss of bone. Inhaled steroids are less likely to cause bone loss than steroids taken by mouth.

- ✓ A baseline BMD with DEXA and evaluation of fracture risk using tools such as FRAX are recommended in all patients who are going to be treated with long term glucocorticoids.

- ✓ Calcitriol is used for preventing glucocorticoid induced bone loss and also post-transplant related bone loss.

- ✓ Bone loss seems to decrease rapidly after discontinuation of glucocorticoid therapy.

- ✓ Glucocorticoids decrease calcium absorption and increase renal calcium excretion; this negative calcium balance leads to secondary hyperparathyroidism and osteoclast activation. Osteoblast activity is directly impaired by glucocorticoids. Steroids also lead to muscle atrophy and decreased muscle strength.

- ✓ In long term glucocorticoid treatment at therapeutic doses, bone loss is likely and should be prevented.

- ✓ If prevention of bone loss is ineffective, treatment is necessary:
    - o Calcium and Vitamin D supplementation.
    - o Antiresorptive therapy with Bisphosphonates is the first choice.
    - o Anabolic therapy with Teriparatide if antiresorptive therapy is unresponsive.

(O) Preventing Falls In Osteoporotic Patients To Avoid Fractures

Each year, about 1/3rd of all people above the age of 65 years, fall. Many of these falls result in broken bones. Some common causes of falls include outdoor and indoor lifestyle behaviours.

Outdoor Safety Tips:

- o Wear low-heeled shoes with rubber soles for more solid footing.
- o Use handrails as you go up and down on escalators.
- o If sidewalks look slippery, walk in the grass for a more solid footing.
- o Use a shoulder bag to leave your hands free so that even if you fall you can take support with your hands.
- o Use a walker or stick if needed.
- o Consider wearing hip protectors or hip pads for added protection.

Indoor Safety Tips:

- o Remove all loose wires, cords.
- o Be sure all carpets and rugs have skid-proof backing.
- o Install grab bars on the bathroom walls beside the tub, shower and toilet.
- o Install sturdy handrails on both sides of stairs.

- Keep a flashlight with fresh batteries beside your bed.
- If you are in a hurry, slow down. Accidents are more likely to happen when you are in a rush.
- Be careful about drinking alcohol.

By using these steps, one can avoid falls, thereby avoiding fractures and can enjoy healthy life.

CHAPTER V: CONCLUSION

"My belief is that it's a prestige to get older. Not everybody gets to get older."

Cameron Diaz

- The biggest achievement in the last century is greater longevity that has resulted in an increasing aged population worldwide.

- Globally average life expectancy has increased from 66.8 years in 2000 to 73.4 years in 2019. But healthy life expectancy has increased from 58.3 in 2000 to 63.7 years in 2019. **In other word healthy life expectancy (5.4 years) is not keeping pace with the increase in life expectancy (6.6 years).**

- The advantage of increased longevity is only when it is translated into healthy ageing.

- It is obvious that women live significant part of their life after menopause.

- It's not correct that women are universally careless about menopausal changes. However some women might not prioritize discussing and addressing menopause due to various reasons such as cultural norms, lack of awareness, discomfort or other priorities.

- Menopause itself is not an illness or medical condition. It is completely a natural ageing event in women's life.

- However the troublesome symptoms that the menopause can bring are frequently unrecognized and undervalued. They are not taken seriously and there are underdiagnosed and undertreated.

- The ovaries after long years of dedicated service, have not the ability of retiring gracefully. But because of estrogen deficiency, ovaries become irritable and transmit this irritation to various organs of the body.

- Many women going through menopause experience unpleasant symptoms such as hot flashes, night sweats, anxiety, depression and poor sleep which can affect their relationship with their spouse.

- Additionally, the risk of non-communicable diseases such as cardiovascular disease, hypertension, diabetes, osteoporosis and cancers increase following menopause.

- Studies have shown that non-communicable diseases affect more women than men globally.

- Because menopause occurs later in life, it is challenging to separate the increased risk of non-communicable diseases due to ageing and increased risk due to menopause. The biology and symptomatology is blurred due to its relationship to the underlying ageing process.

- However several studies have found a correlation between the age that women start menopause and an increased risk of non-communicable diseases. Long term effects on the heart, bone and urogenital system have been related to estrogen deficiency.

- **In this book, I have tried to unravel the facts about heart and bone health in relation to menopause**.

- **In addition to the risks common to both genders, estrogen deficiency in menopause certainly pose additional risk factor in both cardiovascular disease and osteoporosis.**

- **Key points to be noted are:**
    - Menopause is an universal and natural event in women's life.

    - Menopause is inevitable but we can make it easy and equally beautiful by understanding it.

    - Cardiovascular disease (CVD) is number one killer in women especially after menopause, cancer being second.

    - Women can develop heart disease at any age, but the risk increases after menopause, usually after 55 years of age.

    - While average age for heart attack is 64.5 years for men and 70.3 years for women, nearly 20% of those who die of heart disease are under the age of 65 years.

- Studies have shown that estrogen deficiency in menopause is an added risk factor to cardiovascular disease other than the risk factors common to both genders.

- Additionally, there are some nontraditional women-specific risk factors for CVD such as pregnancy complications, polycystic ovarian disease, autoimmune diseases and age at menarche.

- Osteoporosis is not a terminal illness and does not itself directly influence life expectancy. However, having a fracture which is obvious even with a lesser trauma (as the bones are fragile), can definitely affect it.

- Somewhere between the ages of 25 and 35, the rate of bone breakdown will eventually outweigh the rate of bone formation. Bone loss begins to happen at an approximate rate of 0.25% a year and is variable depending upon genetic and environmental factors. This can be attributed as a part of ageing process.

- But menopause significantly speeds up bone loss and increases the risk of osteoporosis. Maximum bone loss occurs between 3-5 years after menopause and after that it slows down. Approximately 1 in 10 women over the age of 60 are affected by osteoporosis worldwide.

What is advisable to reduce the risk of cardiovascular disease and osteoporosis?

- ✓ Every problem has a solution only if we perhaps change our attitude. Women should come out of the age-cage and should redefine age. Women should realize that life after the 4th decade till the end can be more productive if they look after their health, exercise their brain and reinforce the healthy lifestyle changes.

- ✓ The menopause transition or early postmenopause is the **"Window of Opportunity"** to screen and to treat women for menopause related problems, non-communicable diseases and also to detect and treat cancer in early stages, if any, to prevent long-term morbidity due to advanced staging, thus promoting healthy ageing.

- ✓ At menopause clinic, healthcare provider is usually a gynecologist who takes detailed history, does physical examination including breast and pelvic examination, investigates her, identifies risk factors and formulate a plan for individualized counseling and treatment.

- ✓ **Women with non-communicable diseases diagnosed primarily on symptomatology, physical examination and investigations; are referred to respective specialties for better management.**

Lifestyle management for reducing the risk of cardiovascular disease:

By adopting a healthy lifestyle, you can help keep your blood pressure, cholesterol, blood sugars and body weight within normal limits; and lower your risk of heart attacks.

Here are some lifestyle changes that postmenopausal women can adopt to help reduce the risk of cardiovascular disease.

Eat a heart-healthy diet: Focus on consuming a balanced diet rich in fruits, vegetables, whole grains, lean proteins and healthy fats. Limit the intake of saturated and trans fats, sodium and added sugars. Unhealthy fats like saturated and trans fats can raise cholesterol levels and increase the risk of heart disease. Too much sodium can contribute to high blood pressure, which is a risk factor for heart disease. Excessive sugar intake can contribute to weight gain and increase the risk of heart disease. Minimize consumption of desserts and processed snacks. Opt for natural sources of sweetness like fruits.

Maintain healthy weight: Aim for a healthy body weight by incorporating regular physical activity and mindful food choices. Losing excess weight, if necessary, can help reduce the risk of cardiovascular disease. Be mindful of portion sizes to avoid overeating. Use smaller plates and bowls and pay attention to hunger and fullness cues.

Stay physically active: Engage in regular physical activities such as brisk walking, swimming, cycling or dancing. Aim for at least 150 minutes of moderate-intensity or 75 minutes of vigorous-intensity aerobic activity per week along with strength training exercises.

Quit smoking: If you smoke, quitting is one of the most important steps you can take to improve heart health.

Manage Stress: Find healthy ways to manage stress, such as practicing relaxation techniques, engaging in hobbies, spending time with loved ones, or seek professional help if needed. Chronic stress can contribute to cardiovascular disease risk.

Control blood pressure and cholesterol levels: Regularly monitor and manage your blood pressure and cholesterol levels through lifestyle modifications and if necessary, with the medications prescribed by your healthcare provider.

Limit alcohol consumption: If you choose to drink alcohol, do so in moderation. This means up to one drink per day for women.

Stay hydrated: Drink plenty of water throughout the day to maintain proper hydration. Limit sugary cold drinks and excessive caffeine intake.

Get regular check-ups: Schedule regular check-ups with your healthcare provider to monitor your overall health, discuss any concerns and receive appropriate screenings and preventive care.

Consult a doctor: It's important to talk to a healthcare professional for personalized advice and recommendations based on individual health factors.

Lifestyle management for reducing the risk of osteoporosis:

There is no complete cure for osteoporosis. But treatment in time can help to slow or stop the loss of bone density and reduce the risk of fractures. This may include calcium rich diet, calcium and vitamin D supplements, lifestyle changes including exercise, medications if required and steps to prevent fracturing a bone.

Diet: Focus on diet rich in calcium and vitamin D. Foods like dairy products, leafy green vegetables, fortified foods and fatty fish can be beneficial.

Exercise: Engage in weight-bearing exercises like walking, jogging, dancing and resistance training to help improve bone density.

Quit Smoking: If applicable, quitting smoking can contribute to better bone health as well as better overall health.

Limit Alcohol: Limit alcohol intake, as excessive consumption can increase the risk of fracture due to fall.

Healthy Weight: Maintain a healthy weight, as being underweight can increase the risk of osteoporosis.

Consult a doctor: It's important to talk to a healthcare professional for personalized advice and recommendations based on individual health factors.

By delving into the multifaceted factors influencing both heart and bone health, this book underscores the need for holistic approaches to women's wellbeing during the postmenopausal phase. The insights garnered here not only contribute to the existing body of knowledge but also hold practical implications for healthcare practitioners, policy makers and women themselves.

In closing, the book **“Postmenopausal Heart and Bone Health”** serves as a stepping stone towards a more comprehensive understanding of the intricate relationship between menopause and heart and bone health. It is my hope that this book ignites ongoing discussions and encourages continued research that ultimately benefits the well-being of postmenopausal women around the world.

CHAPTER VI: REFERENCES

- Clinical Practice on menopause – Indian Menopause Society.
- Journal of Mid Life Health.
- Dinnerstein L, Dudley EC, Hopper JL et. al. A prospective population-based study of menopause symptoms. Obstet. Gynecol 2000; 96:351.
- Woods NF, Mitchell ES. Symptoms during the menopause: prevalence, severity and significance in women's lives. Am J Med 2005; 118 suppl 12 B: 14.
- National Institute of Health State-of-the-Science Conference Statement: management of menopause-related symptoms. Ann Intern Med 2005; 142:1003.
- Kronenberg F. Hot flashes: epidemiology and physiology. Ann N Y Acad Sci 1090; 592:52.
- McKinley SM. The normal menopause transition: an overview. Maturitas 1996; 23:137.
- Cohen LS, Soars CN, Joffe H. Diagnosis and management of mood disorders during menopause transition. Am J Med 2005; 118 suppl 12B:93.
- Freedom RR, Roehrs TA. Sleep disturbances in menopause. Menopause 2007; 14:826.

- Mathews KA, Wings RR, Kuller LH, et.al. Influence of the perimenopause on cardiovascular risk factors and symptoms middle-aged healthy women. Arch Intern Med 1994; 154:2349.

- Thurston RC, Joffe H. Vasomotor symptoms and menopause: findings from the study of women's health across the nation. Obstet. Gynecol Clin North Am 2011; 38:489.

- Mohyi D, Tabassi K, Simon J. Differential diagnosis of hot flashes. Maturitas 1997; 27:203.

- Anklesaria BS. Why should it be the stage of menopause? Modern management of menopause with isoflavones; 2007.PP. 7-9.

- Anklesaria BS. Staging of Menopause. The Menopause FOGSI Focus; 2010. PP. 3 – 5.
- Harlow SD, Gass M, Hall JE, et.al. Executive summary of the stages of reproductive aging workshop + 10: addressing the unfinished agenda of staging reproductive aging. Fertil Steril. 2012;97(4):843-51.

- Brown WJ, Mishra GD, Dobson A. Changes in physical symptoms during the menopause transition. Int J Behav Med 2002;9(1):53-67.

- Barton DL, Loprinzi C, Atherton PJ, et. al. Dehydroepiandrosterone for the treatment of hot flashes: A pilot study. Support cancer then 2006;3(2):91-7.

- Calleja-Agius J, Brincat M. Urogenital atrophy. Climacteric 2009; 12:279-285.

- MacBride M, Rhodes D, Shuster L. Vulvovaginal atrophy. Mayo Clin Proc 2010; 85:87-94.

- Portman D, Gass M, Vulvovaginal Atrophy Terminology Consensus Conference Panel. Genitourinary Syndrome of Menopause: new terminology of vulvovaginal atrophy from International Society for the Study of Women's Sexual Health and the North American Menopause Society. Menopause 2014;21(10);1063-1068.

- Palacios S. Managing urogenital atrophy. Maturitas 2009;63(4):315-318.

- Lester J, Pahouja G, Aderson B, Lustberg M. Atrophic vaginitis in breast cancer survivors: a difficult survivorship issue. J Pers Med 2015;5(2):50-66.

- NICE. Menopause: diagnosis and management of genitourinary syndrome of menopause. NICE Guidelines 23. NICE, 2015. Available at: www.nice.org.uk/ng23.

- Therapies for the management of genitourinary syndrome of menopause. Palacios S, Combalia J, Emsellem C, Gaslain Y, Khorsandi D. Post Repro Health. 2020;26:32-42. (Pubmed) (Google Scholar).

- ACOG Practice Bulletin No. 141: management of menopausal symptoms. American College of Obstetrician and Gynaecologist. Obstet Gynecol. 2014;123:202-216, (Pubmed) (Google Scholar).

- Genitourinary changes with aging. Mitchell CM, Waetjen LE. Obstet Gynecol Clin North Am. 2018;45:737-750. (Pubmed) (Google Scholar).

- The role of local vaginal oestrogen for treatment of vaginal atrophy in postmenopausal women:2007 position statement of the North American Society. Menopause 2007;14:355-369. (Pubmed) (Google Scholar).

- Genitourinary Syndrome of Menopause: common problem, effective treatments. Phillips NA, Bachmann GA. Cleve Clin J Med. 2018;85:390-398. (Pubmed) (Google Scholar).

- Genitourinary Syndrome of menopause. Briggs P. Post Report Health. 2019:2053369119884144. (PubMed) (Google Scholar).

- Genitourinary syndrome of menopause: an overview of clinical manifestations, pathophysiology, aetiology, evaluation and management. Gandhi J, Chen A, Dagur G, Suh Y, Smit N, Cali B, Khan SA, Am J Obstet Gynecol. 2016;215:504-711. (PubMed) (Google Scholar).

- Yasuda H. RANKL, a necessary chance for clinical application to osteoporosis and cancer-related bone disease. World J Orthop. 2013;4:207-217.(PMC free article) (PubMed) (Google Scholar).

- Sambrook P, Cooper C. Osteoporosis. Lancet. 2006;368:2010-2018 (Pub Med) (Google Scholar).

- Rossini M, Adami S, Bertoldo F, et.al. Guidelines for the diagnosis, prevention and management of osteoporosis. Reumatismo. 2016;68:1-39. (PubMed) (Google Scholar).

- Bauer JS, Link TM. Advances in osteoporosis imaging. Europ J Radiol. 2009;71:440-449 (PubMed) (Google Scholar).

- National Osteoporosis Foundation, 2013 Clinician's Guide for prevention and treatment of osteoporosis. http://nof/public/contenr/resource/913/files/580.pdf (Accepted on November 14, 2013).

- American Association of Clinical Endocrinologists Medical Guidelines for clinical practice for the diagnosis and treatment of postmenopausal osteoporosis.

- Global AL, Laya MB (May 2015), "Osteoporosis: screening, prevention and management." The Medical Clinics of North America. 99(3):587-606. Doi:10. 1016/j.mcna. 2015.01.010. PMID 25841602.

- Clinical Challenges: Managing osteoporosis in male hypogonadism. www.medpagetoday.com. 4 June 2018. Retrieved 22 March 2022.

- Rigo J, et.al Reference values of body composition obtained by dual x-ray absorptiometry in preterm and term neonates. J Pediatr Gastroenterol Nutr. 1998;27:184-90. (PubMed) (Google Scholar).

- Hlaing TT, Compston JE. Biochemical markers of bone turnover-uses and limitations. Ann Clin Biochem 2014; 51:189.

- Bauer D, Krege J, Lane N, et.al. National Bone Health Alliance Bone Turnover Marker Project: current practices and the need for US harmonization, standardization and common reference ranges. Osteoporosis Int 2012;23:2425.

- The NAMS 2017 Hormone Therapy Position Statement Advisory Panel. The 2017 hormone therapy position statement of the North American Menopause Society. Menopause 2017;24:728.

- Steingold KA, Laufer L, Chetkowski RJ, et.al. Treatment of hot flashes with transdermal estradiol administration. J Clin Endocrinol Metab 1985;61:627.

- Nelson HD. Commonly used types of postmenopausal oestrogen for treatment of hot flashes: scientific review. JAWA 2004; 291:1610.

- North American Menopause Society. The 2012 hormone position statement of: The North American Menopause Society. Menopause 2012;19:257.

- Sood R, Faubion SS, Kuhle CL et.al prescribing Menopause Therapy: an evidence-based approach. Int. J Women's Health 2014;6:47.

- Udoff L, Langenberg P, Adashi EY. Combined Continuous Hormone Replacement Therapy: a critical review. Obstet Gynecol 1995;86:306.

- ACOG Practice Bulletin No. 141: management of menopausal symptoms. Obstet Gynecol. 2014;123(1):202-216.

- Bakour SH, Williamson J. Latest evidence on using hormone therapy in the menopause. Obstet Gynecol, 2014.

- The 2022 hormone therapy position statement of the North American Menopause Society. Menopause (New York). 2022;29(7):767-794.

- Lee MH, Kim SH, Oh M, Lee KW, Park MJ. Age at menarche in Korean adolescents: trends and influencing factors. *Reprod Health.* 2016; 13:121. (PMC free article) (PubMed) (Google Scholar)

- Lim JS, Lee HS, Kim EY, Yi KH, Hwang JS. Early menarche increases the risk of type 2 diabetes in young and middle aged Korean woman. *Diabet Med.* 2015; 32:521-5. (PubMed) (Google Scholar).

- Kessous R, Shoham-Vardi I, Pariente G, Shef M, Sheiner E. An association between gestational diabetes mellitus and long-term cardiovascular morbidity. Heart (2013) 99:1118-21. Doi: 10.1136/heartjnl-2013-303945.

- Goueslard K, Collenet J, Mariet A-S, Giroud M, Cottin Y, Petit JM, et al. Early cardiovascular events in women with a history of gestational diabetes. *Cardiovac Diabetol* (2016) 15:15. Doi: 10.1186/s12933-016-0338-0

- Carr DB, Utzschneider, KM, Hull RL, Tong J, Wallace TM, Kodama K et.al. Gestational diabetes mellitus increases the risk of cardiovascular disease in women with a family history of type 2 diabetes. *Diabetes care* (2006) 29:2078-83. Doi: 10.2337/dc05-2482

- Lauenborg J, Matheiesen E, Hansen T, Glumer C, Jorgensen T, Borch-Johsen K, et.al. The prevalence of the metabolic syndrome in a Danish population of women with previous gestational diabetes mellitus is three-fold higher than the general population. *J Clin Endocrinol Metab* (2005) 90:4004-10. Doi:10.1210/jc.2004-1713

- Blencowe H, Cousen S, Chou D, Oestergaad M, Say L,Mller AB, Kinney M, Lawn J. Born too soon: the global epidemiology of million preterm births. **Reprod Health**. 2013; 10:S2. **Google Scholar**

- Heida KY, Velthuis BK, Oudijk MA, Reitsma JB, Bot ML, Franx A, Van Dunne FM. Cardiovascular disease risk in women with a history of spontaneous preterm delivery: a systematic review and meta-analysis. **Eur J Prev Cardiol.** 2015; 23:253-263. **Google Scholar**.

- Robbins CL, Hutchings Y, Dietz PM, Kuklina EV, Callaghan WM. History of preterm birth and subsequent cardiovascular disease: a systematic review. **Am J Obstet Gyneco**l. 2014; 210:285-297. **Google Scholar.**

- B. Leanne, C. Juan-Pablo, A.D. Hingorani, D.J. Williams Pre-eclampsia disease and cancer in later life: systemic review and meta-analysis. BMJ Br Med J (Clin Res Ed), 335 (2007), pp. 974-977 **Google Scholar.**

- W.B. LDK Patterns of coronary heart disease morbidity and mortality in the sexes: a 26-years follow-up of the Framingham population. Am Heart J, 111 (2) (1986), PP. 383-390. **Google Scholar.**

- P. Appelros, B. Stegmayr, A. Terent Sex differences in stroke epidemiology: a systematic review. Stroke, 40 (2009), pp. 1082-1090. **Google Scholar.**

Previous books written in the series "Women's Health"

1. Preconception Care makes a difference

The link is given below:

w.amazon.com/s?k=Preconception+care+makes+a+difference+book+by+dinesh+kanfade&crid=1LD9L1M6MLOWA&sprefix=preconception+care+makes+a+differ

2. Understanding Menopause

The link is given below:

https://www.amazon.com/gp/product/B0C6FJ6XN8?ref_=dbs_m_mng_rwt_calw_tkin_1&storeType=ebooks&qid=1693134113&sr=8-2

www.ingramcontent.com/pod-product-compliance
Lightning Source LLC
LaVergne TN
LVHW021139160826
845679LV00023B/1968

9798891330672